Continuing Professional Development
Development
A Guide for Therapists

Auldeen Alsop
MPhil, BA, DipCOT, MHSM

Blackwell
Science

© 2000 by Blackwell Science Ltd, a Blackwell Publishing Company
Editorial Offices:
Blackwell Science Ltd, 9600 Garsington Road, Oxford OX4 2DQ, UK
  Tel: +44 (0)1865 776868
Blackwell Publishing Inc., 350 Main Street, Malden, MA 02148-5020, USA
  Tel: +1 781 388 8250
Blackwell Science Asia Pty Ltd, 550 Swanston Street, Carlton, Victoria 3053, Australia
  Tel: +61 (0)3 8359 1011

First published 2000
Reprinted 2001, 2003, 2004

Library of Congress Cataloging-in-Publication Data
Alsop, Auldeen
   Continuing professional development : a guide for therapists / Auldeen Alsop
       p.   cm.
   Includes bibliographical references and index
   ISBN 0-632-05007-1 (pb)
   1. Occupational therapy—Study and teaching (Continuing education).   I. Title.
   [DNLM: 1. Occupational therapy—education.   2. Education, Continuing.
   3. Professional Competence. WB 18
   A462c 2000]
   RM735.42.A465 2000
   615.8′515′0715—dc21

                                                                    99-059642

ISBN 0-632-05007-1

A catalogue record for this title is available from the British Library

Set in 10/12.5pt Century Book
by DP Photosetting, Aylesbury, Bucks
Printed and bound in Great Britain
by Marston Book Services, Oxford

The publisher's policy is to use permanent paper from mills that operate a sustainable forestry policy, and which has been manufactured from pulp processed using acid-free and elementary chlorine-free practices. Furthermore, the publisher ensures that the text paper and cover board used have met acceptable environmental accreditation standards.

For further information on Blackwell Publishing, visit our website:
www.blackwellpublishing.com

Contents

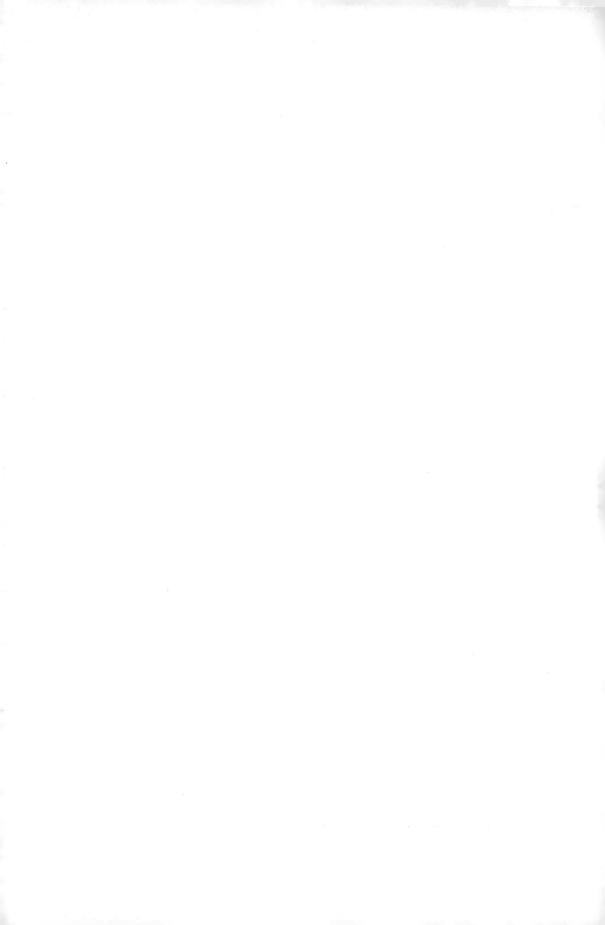

Foreword

'Lifelong learning is a continuous development process which can be said to belong to an individual'

(Teare *et al.*, 1998).

Successive governments have made lifelong learning a major policy objective, and there have been many studies of the subject. But at the same time that the government is introducing the concept of lifelong learning to health and social care practitioners, it also has to ensure that statutory obligations to the patient are fulfilled. In May 1996 the General Medical Council stated:

'We are committed to a system of medical revelation which is open and accountable and to developing procedures and processes that are effective, fair, objective, transparent and free from discriminations'.

Practitioners have to be aware that the government expects individuals to be responsible for the quality of their own clinical practice. Auldeen Alsop's timely book deals with the link between lifelong learning and ensuring that practitioners are equipped to operate in a safe and professional manner.

Health care practitioners often have to grapple with a balance between theory and practice. This book unpicks some of the commonly-used theoretical phrases such as criteria of competence and portfolio generation, and applies them to practice in a wide variety of settings. Within a busy practice environment it enables practitioners to formulate a way in which they can ensure that they both keep up to date and continue to enhance their skills and gain qualifications in ways which are flexible and appropriate to their learning skills and lifestyles.

Auldeen Alsop has provided a comprehensive book on continuing professional development which all practitioners will find of benefit, whether they just choose to read one or two chapters or whether they look further into the background and mechanisms of continuing professional development. Each chapter concludes with a set of references for further reading and with practical suggestions to ensure that development is reflected upon and achievements noted.

Auldeen indicates that this book is designed to help any practitioner along the professional journey, and hopes that it will help many to realise their dreams: I am confident that it will.

Dawn Forman
MBA, PGDip Research Methods, MDCR, TDCR
Dean of School of Health and Community Studies
University of Derby

Reference

Teare, R., Davies, D. & Sandelands, E. (1998) *The Virtual University in Action: Paradigm and Process for Workplace Learning*. London, Cassells.

Preface

In our journey through life from birth to old age we engage constantly in different learning experiences that together equip us to look after ourselves, to engage effectively in society and to cope with the changing circumstances around us. These lifelong learning experiences provide us with insights about ourselves and others, help us to develop a store of knowledge and skills to draw on when needed, and assist us to prepare for and manage the challenges associated with different life stages.

This book is primarily concerned with challenges between studenthood and retirement. It relates most particularly to learning and continuing professional development during a health professional's career after initial professional qualification. The key issue is continuing professional development for the purpose of competence maintenance, although competence enhancement and competence development feature widely. Currently, continuing professional development is a voluntary activity that should benefit the individual undertaking it, the organisation in which he or she works and, above all, the users of the services provided. The ongoing engagement of practitioners in learning and professional development also provides an assurance to the public of continued professional competence.

There was a view, confirmed by JM Consulting (1996), that measures more stringent than those provided under the Professions Supplementary to Medicine Act 1960 were needed to ensure protection of the public. A framework was needed within which each state registered practitioner should take steps to maintain competence to practise in his or her profession. This would entail each individual taking responsibility for his or her ongoing learning and for being able to provide the evidence that steps were being taken to update knowledge and skills and thus to maintain competence to practise. Under the new Health Act 1999 there is provision for the assessment of this continued competence and for steps to be taken where there is concern about the adequacy of a professional's competence in professional practice.

Everyone involved in health and social care provision is well aware that the practice world is constantly changing. We live in an environment where dynamic sociological, political and economic factors have a major impact on what we do. As they change, so practice changes. We have to stay in tune with the nature of practice and its wider environment in order to understand health care provision, the direction that it is taking and the consequences for ourselves as health care professionals.

One of the more recent changes proposed in the Government's White Paper, *The New NHS: modern, dependable* (1997), is the concept of clinical governance. This concept and its impact will be explored later in the book, but the White Paper clearly stated (p. 59) that the Government will look to individual health professionals to be responsible for the quality of their own clinical practice. Maintaining quality in practice involves keeping up to date with practice and applying the evidence base for practice to the work situation. Taking responsibility for maintaining competence and thus the quality of practice must therefore be built into the route that we take through our professional career. Maintaining competence and striving to improve our professional performance is essential, a non-negotiable aspect of our practice. How we do it is largely up to us.

We chose our profession because of the personal rewards that we anticipated from engaging in the activity associated with it. Professional activity has to be enjoyable for it to be sustained. Learning, developing and growing as a professional person, and in the process of being professional, has to be enjoyable too. Learning is integral to practice, not disassociated from it, but we need to know that it is leading somewhere if it is to be planned and pursued. Learning also has to be ongoing and part of the vision of where we see ourselves on our journey in the future. Knowles (1990, p. 32) cites Jacks (1929) in this respect:

> 'Earning and living are not two separate departments or operations in life. They are two names for a continuous process looked at from opposite ends . . . Education based on this vision of *continuity* is the outstanding need of our times. Its outlook will be lifelong. It will look upon the industry of civilisation as the great "continuation school" for intelligence and for character, and its object will be, not merely to fit men and women for the specialised vocations they are to follow, but also to animate the vocations themselves with ideals of excellence appropriate to each.'

This was true vision, a dream that lifelong learning within society and for society would be the essence of personal growth 'with ideals of excellence' guiding us in earning, living and learning.

In a short article Karen Jacobs, newly appointed president of the American Occupational Therapy Association, wrote about her dreams (1998). 'Dreams are my vision' she said, 'where I want to end up'. 'A dreamer looks beyond the limits of today to the possibility of tomorrow'. Referring to Pitino & Reynolds (1997) Jacobs suggested that success, not just in dreams but in reality, means building self-esteem, setting demanding goals, always being positive, establishing good habits, mastering the art of communication, learning from role models, thriving on pressure, being persistent, learning from adversity and surviving success. Learning and continuing to develop professionally have to be identified with a vision that not only ensures ongoing competence to practise but also takes us further on the journey through professional life to where *we* want to end up.

References

Jacks, L.P. (1929) *Journal of Adult Education* **1**, 7–10.

Jacobs, K. (1998) Harnessing your dreams. *OT Week* 12 (32), 7.

JM Consulting Ltd (1996) *The Regulation of Health Professions*. Department of Health, London.

Knowles, M. (1990) *Adult Learner a Neglected Species*, 4th edn. Gulf Publishing Company, Houston.

Pitino, R. & Reynolds, B. (1997) *Success is a Choice*. Broadway Books, New York.

The New NHS – Modern, Dependable (1997) The Stationery Office, London.

Chapter 1
Continuing Professional Development

Some definitions

Continuing professional development (CPD) is a term commonly used to denote the process of the ongoing education and development of health care professionals, from initial qualifying education and for the duration of professional life, in order to maintain competence to practise and increase professional proficiency and expertise. Many organisations seem to have attempted to define continuing professional development and, although there are slight variations in the definitions, the underlying message is fairly consistent. The Chartered Society of Physiotherapy (CSP) (1996), for example, defined continuing professional development succinctly as:

> 'an educational process by which professional people maintain, enhance and broaden professional competence'.

We note particularly the words 'educational process' since Eraut (1994) argued that CPD is wider than just *education*. He made the distinction between continuing professional education (CPE) and continuing professional development. Continuing professional education, he maintained, includes formal study programmes, courses or conferences that individuals attend, whereas continuing professional development (CPD) embraces many other activities through which individuals learn and develop their skills and expertise. It includes informal learning and on-the-job learning and can also include forms of both intended and incidental learning, a theme explored later in this book. Nevertheless, all CPD involves learning and in that respect it could be viewed as an educational process.

In an unpublished consultation paper for the Chartered Society of Physiotherapy, Powell (1997) suggested that continuing professional development should provide assurance of competence in practice and be measured in a way that shows a demonstrable impact on health outcomes. This implies that there should be a direct relationship between continuing professional development and the effectiveness of health care. The definition of continuing professional development in the Government's document *A First Class Service* reinforced this (Department of Health, 1998, p. 84). It described CPD as 'a process of lifelong learning for all individuals and teams that meets the needs of patients and delivers the health outcomes and health care priorities of the NHS and that enables professionals to expand and fulfil their potential'. Although there currently seems to be little evidence that improved health outcomes are directly associated with professional development, the later document on continuing professional development (Department of Health, 1999) made explicit how this should happen, linking CPD to the clinical governance agenda.

The College of Occupational Therapists (1994) referred to continuing professional development as a career-long process that builds on what the practitioner already knows and prepares him or her for changing roles in service delivery. This definition can be seen as being in tune with the concept of enabling the expansion and fulfilment of potential. It also suggests that it is a mechanism that enables services to meet the needs of their users in a changing health care environment. These definitions can be linked. Service delivery in health care has to be concerned with effectiveness and therefore with beneficial health outcomes for service users. The capacity of practitioners both to maintain competence and to modify what they do in line with changing circumstances is crucial to the process.

The definition of CPD endorsed in *Continuing Professional Development: Quality in the New NHS* (Department of Health, 1999) embraces the concept of lifelong learning for all health professionals as an investment in quality. A more general, but seemingly widely accepted definition of CPD is one coined initially by the construction industry and adopted by the Local Government Management Board (1993) and the Institute of Continuing Professional Development. In its promotional literature the Institute defined CPD as:

> 'the systematic maintenance, improvement and broadening of knowledge and skill and the development of personal qualities necessary for the execution of professional and technical duties throughout the practitioner's working life'.

This reiterates the CSP definition with an emphasis on the systematic nature of the process of CPD. It suggests that CPD needs to be planned and structured and should not be left to chance. One further definition offered by the Institute of Continuing Professional Development was:

> 'a process by which a professional person maintains the quality and relevance of professional services throughout his/her working life'.

Again, this stresses that CPD is a long-term process rather than an end product, but also states that it has a specific purpose directly related to the quality of service provision.

These particular definitions address the personal qualities of the practitioner and also acknowledge both the technical and professional facets of practice that need to be developed. All definitions see continuing professional development as a long-term process spanning the full period of a professional's career. If we accept that this is so, then we need to pay attention to the process in whatever post we hold and throughout all the changes that we make in employment or our professional career.

So perhaps the dimensions and expectations of continuing professional development can now be summarised as the following:

- A process (rather than a product)
- Lifelong, ongoing throughout professional life
- Systematic
- Embracing formal education and informal learning, including on-the-job learning
- Building on what is known, in order to
  - Assure competence
  - Develop personal qualities
  - Enhance professional and technical skills
  - Maintain, enhance and broaden professional knowledge
  - Expand and help fulfil potential
  - Have a positive impact on health outcomes
  - Maintain quality and relevance of professional services
  - Develop and enhance practice
  - Prepare for changing roles in service delivery

Continuing professional development is thus concerned both with the individual and with the service and with quality of professional performance both currently and in the future. References in some professional literature also expect CPD to lead to improved service quality and value for money. So, linking the various definitions we might conclude that the purpose of CPD is to ensure competent practice that will maximise the potential and the professional performance of the therapist, minimise risk to service users and lead to improvements in service efficiency and effectiveness.

Continuing professional development and the individual

Continuing professional development has to be at the heart of each professional's practice to enable practitioners, not only to remain competent, but also to develop and grow and so to fulfil their potential at all stages of their professional career. CPD can be planned in order to facilitate professional growth or it can emerge through different experiences in professional life. These experiences have to be revisited, reviewed systematically and then translated, through reflection and evaluation, into learning. They can then be stored and drawn upon in current practice or used later to inform future developments. Continuing professional development is thus seen as an individual professional's responsibility and this is often made explicit in a profession's Code of Conduct. Once qualified, each professional has a duty to maintain a state of competence so that he or she can practise with due regard for public safety and well-being and ensure that cost-effective and up-to-date interventions are used in practice. Quality initiatives (Department of Health, 1998) to support the new NHS stress that health care professionals must be accountable for their own practice, and this includes updating practice in order to maintain professional standards and standards of patient care.

It has been noted that continuing professional development is an ongoing process throughout a professional's career but there is a distinct difference between the responsibilities and the experience of initial professional education and continuing professional education and development. Unlike skills and competent performance that are initially developed through a defined pre-registration qualifying programme, CPD has to be self-initiated and self-directed. Learning must be planned and negotiated personally rather than being structured and assessed by others. Judgements about personal competence formerly undertaken by other people have to be built into professional practice as self-evaluation of a practitioner's own performance. This shift from engaging in a structured programme to devising and implementing a personal learning strategy can be difficult. Many practitioners will not be well-versed in the process of monitoring and evaluating their own performance, setting their own learning agenda and organising their study time. Many degree programmes leading to professional qualifications now enable students to recognise how learning occurs. They encourage student practitioners to develop their learning skills and to become self-directed in the process of learning. Somehow this is not always enough as other responsibilities take priority when the newly qualified practitioner starts work. Managing a workload, managing learning and integrating learning systematically into professional life is not easy. It takes time, self-discipline and good personal organisation. In order to commit to continuing professional development professionals have to see the potential benefits of this activity and then develop the skills to ensure that learning and professional development become integral to practice and not just an adjunct to it.

Personal benefits

Regardless of any statutory requirements for professionals to take steps to remain competent, every professional should see the personal benefits to be gained from engaging in development activity. CPD will only be of real benefit if the learning takes place as a voluntary activity, as part of a process of lifelong learning and as part of a personal commitment to self-development. No amount of legislation on CPD will ever ensure that learning will support competent practice unless the individual him or herself actually wishes to learn. This means that CPD activity needs to be meaningful for an individual if it is to be taken seriously and the benefits to the individual need to be clear and to be valued. There are undoubtedly costs attached, not least in terms of time commitment, so benefits must be identified in order to provide the motivation to pursue relevant development activity. Continuing professional development can be thought to have many benefits. For example, it

- Encourages a higher standard of personal professional performance
- Demonstrates commitment to best practice
- Demonstrates commitment to service users
- Demonstrates commitment to current and future employers
- Offers increased job satisfaction
- Provides the means to anticipate, plan and prepare for change
- Enhances professional knowledge, skills and status
- Promotes awareness of new developments and concepts
- Expands areas of expertise
- Improves personal efficiency
- Provides a framework for making informed decisions about future professional activity
- Offers the means of improving career prospects and taking on new roles
- Provides opportunity for making new contacts through CPD activity and for developing a network of people with similar skills and interests

Any one of these reasons should provide sufficient grounds for contemplating and engaging in continuing professional development, irrespective of any statutory obligation or framework that formalises the requirements.

Statutory provision

A review by JM Consulting Ltd (1996) of the Professions Supplementary to Medicine Act 1960 highlighted the deficiencies in the legislation, noting particularly the absence of any expectation regarding continuing competence or continuing professional development for those state registered under the Act. Provisions under the Health Act 1999 allow for the monitoring of the education and training of health professionals before and after their admission to practice. In this respect, state registered practitioners wishing to retain their name on the register, and those desiring to re-register after a break in service, are likely to have to demonstrate their continuing competence to practise in their profession.

Although the Health Act 1999 is intended to serve the same main function as the 1960 Act with regard to the protection of the public, the emphasis is on improvement in the quality of health care. Various mechanisms are to be introduced to promote and oversee improvements and to deal with inadequate performance at individual and organisational level. Each professional will thus need to provide evidence of his or her continued competence to practise. Individuals who take a systematic approach to CPD will readily be able to demonstrate the maintenance of their competence as a fundamental requirement of continued state registration. Those who are interested in career advancement or in the development of their expertise can work beyond the basic requirements to show how their competence is developing in both breadth and depth as preparation for new roles in health care.

Continuing professional development and health care

The Government's clear intention is to improve health care through clinical governance and continuing professional development. The document *Continuing Professional Development: Quality in the New NHS* (Department of Health, 1999) linked CPD to standards of health care and promoted CPD as a shared responsibility between the employing organisation and the individual. It stated that 'continuing professional development should be a partnership between the individual and the organisation, its focus should be on the delivery of high quality NHS services as well as meeting individual career aspirations and learning needs' (p. 4). The document went on to suggest that CPD 'should meet the wider service development needs of the NHS and that employers should value CPD as an integral part of quality improvement' (p. 8). It reconfirmed appraisal as 'the cornerstone' of assessing the CPD needed for each individual and personal development plans (PDPs) as the process through which CPD would be implemented to align with organisational needs (p. 11). CPD plans should not just promote individual learning and development but team learning for practice development.

Of course not all healthcare practitioners will be National Health Service employees. Some may work as private practitioners, others for the independent sector, charitable services or for another public service such as social services. The principles of CPD as outlined in the Department of Health (1999) document could still be seen as underpinning effective practice in whatever organisation health practitioners are employed. The Department of Health (1999, p. 6) noted that organisations accredited as Investors in People would already have PDPs in place for all staff so it seems that this model is one to be promoted. Individuals who take seriously their responsibility and take steps to maintain the knowledge and skills needed for professional practice, wherever they work, will enhance their ability to move between different parts of the service both within the employing organisation and between different employing organisations.

The process of continuing professional development

The process of continuing professional development can take a number of forms dependent on whether the focus for the individual is on personal career development or on maintaining and developing knowledge and skills to underpin competent performance in the current job. It is not that these are necessarily incompatible, but the first will take a broad, longer term and personal view whereas the second will be focused on shorter term needs prompted by performance review and related largely to service provision. The process of CPD is much the same as any other process designed to bring about change and improvement, for example, the therapeutic process or audit process. The CPD process similarly involves:

- assessing need
- defining the goals
- planning to attain the goals
- implementing the plan
- evaluating the effectiveness of the process
- reviewing need and redefining the plan.

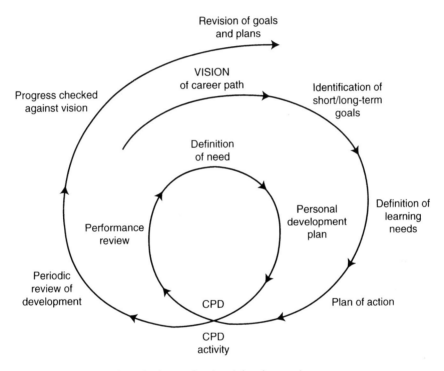

Fig. 1.1 The process of continuing professional development.

These stages are illustrated in the CPD cycle shown in Fig. 1.1. The diagram shows the interrelationship between career development activity (outer cycle) and service-related CPD activity identified in personal development plans (inner cycle). Vision, or a view of the future, is necessary for both, and CPD activity is integrated into both cycles, supporting both sets of plans. At the end of the cycle, it is obviously important to know whether the planned CPD activity was successful in meeting the defined goals and where subsequent effort should be directed. A revised view of needs and goals has to be formed to reflect personal, professional, organisational and environmental changes that have occurred, and plans must be updated to reflect ongoing need. It is a process that should indicate where a change in level and application of knowledge has led to desired outcomes, personally, professionally and, as appropriate, service-related.

Chapter 4 further discusses the short and long term professional development needs in relation to a practitioner's current role and career aspirations. Records of achievement and evidence of competence maintenance and development emerging from the professional development process are likely to be compiled into portfolio form. The next chapter explores how a portfolio can be used for this purpose.

References

Chartered Society of Physiotherapy (1996) *CPD: Guidelines of Good Practice for Physiotherapists, Managers and Educators.* Information Paper Number CPD 4. Chartered Society of Physiotherapy, London.

College of Occupational Therapists (1994) *Post-qualifying Guidance and Directory.* College of Occupational Therapists, London.

Department of Health (1998) *A First Class Service – Quality in the New NHS.* Department of Health, Leeds.

Department of Health (1999) *Continuing Professional Development: Quality in the New NHS.* Department of Health, Leeds.

Eraut, M. (1994) *Developing Professional Knowledge and Competence.* The Falmer Press, London.

JM Consulting Ltd (1996) *The Regulation of Health Professions.* Department of Health, London.

Local Government Management Board (1993) *Continuing Professional Development – Partnership for Change.* The Local Government Management Board, Luton.

Powell, A. (1997) *A Framework for Continuing Professional Development.* Chartered Society of Physiotherapy, London.

Chapter 2
Using Portfolios for Continuing Professional Development

What is a portfolio?

Increasingly there is the expectation that health professionals demonstrate that they have engaged in the process of learning and continuing professional development, so there has to be some means of presenting evidence of this. It is commonly recommended that the evidence of CPD be collected and presented in portfolio form. But what is a portfolio and how should it be used?

One of the original uses of a portfolio was for presenting examples of an artist's work to show evidence of the range and quality of an individual's work and capability for employment. The word 'portfolio' is derived from the Latin *portare* meaning 'to carry' and *folium* meaning 'a leaf' (Alsop, 1995) and is now commonly defined as a 'collection of papers' (Chambers Concise Dictionary) or as a 'collection of papers or artefacts' (Brown & Knight, 1994). The term portfolio has since come to have a wider application in education (Brown & Knight, 1994) and in business marketing (Cannon, 1992), although the primary concept is the same – it is a record of what the portfolio holder has to offer clients.

In simple terms, Redman (1994) tells us that portfolios are concerned with evidence of good practice. Taken a step further, good practice might be said to equate with competent practice. Thus an individual who can show that he or she is currently engaging in good practice, that is, using up-to-date interventions for which there is evidence of their effectiveness and being able to justify their use, is demonstrating his or her continuing professional competence.

The College of Occupational Therapists (1994) described a portfolio as a document in which practitioners can record learning experiences, their evaluation of them and the learning outcomes that have resulted from the learning experiences. Calman (1998) suggested that a portfolio is a personal professional development tool aimed at encouraging reflection and self-direction in identifying training needs. Portfolios record learning opportunities and provide tangible evidence of outcomes. A portfolio is therefore dynamic in that it needs to be updated to reflect ongoing learning needs and opportunities. Similarly, Redman advises us that a portfolio 'is not a historical record of achievement nor a current profile of competence but a living, growing collection of evidence that mirrors the growth of its owner, including his or her hopes and plans for the future' (1994,

p. 42). A portfolio is therefore not merely a curriculum vitae of the owner, nor a list of professional activities, courses or conferences attended, but it is a systematic, documented record of the processes and outcomes of learning showing what has been achieved and how new learning will inform future practice. As Redman therefore suggested, a portfolio is as much about the future as it is about the present and past. Brown captured the essence of this when she defined a portfolio as:

> 'a collection of evidence which demonstrates the continuing acquisition of skills, knowledge, attitudes, understanding and achievement. It is both retrospective and prospective as well as reflecting the current stage of development and activity of the individual'. (1992, p. 1)

Brown and Knight (1994) saw a portfolio not as a heap of everything that comes to hand but as a carefully selected range of artefacts that shows progression and demonstrates improvement over time (p. 82). They affirmed that a critical account of the contents is needed to contextualise the work and to demonstrate learning achieved. It is noticeable in the literature about portfolios that some of the authors make a point of stating very clearly what a portfolio *is not*. We need, however, to come to some conclusion about what a portfolio *is*. Teasing out the elements of the various definitions, it is possible to identify and summarise the attributes or characteristics of a portfolio as:

- A collection of various kinds of material that together serve as an ongoing living record of progress and achievement
- Evidence of acquired knowledge, skills and understanding that demonstrate good practice
- Reflections of past and present activities and experiences that have resulted in and demonstrate learning
- Key features of a professional career that indicate personal growth and professional development
- Details of future plans, goals and a strategy for their attainment
- A critical account of the 'contents' to contextualise the work and demonstrate improvements over time

The list provides a useful guide for selecting, preparing and presenting material and structuring it in portfolio form.

Profiles, portfolios and diaries

It might be helpful at this stage to examine the difference between a profile and portfolio. Professions such as nursing use the term 'profiling'. Since 1995 the United Kingdom Council for Nursing, Midwifery and Health Visiting has required individuals on the professional register to use a Personal Professional Profile as a requirement for continued registration (Hull & Redfern, 1996).

Brown (1992) helpfully distinguished between the two terms by stating that a *profile* is a collection of evidence that is selected from a *portfolio* for a particular purpose and for the attention of a particular audience. A portfolio therefore contains a wider range of references and evidence from which an informed choice of material can be made to be presented as a profile of the individual for a particular purpose. 'Portfolio' is the term that has been taken into common usage by many of the professions allied to medicine and is the term referred to in this book. However, the Chartered Society of Physiotherapy (1994) recommended to its members that they keep a Professional Development Diary for recording and monitoring their professional development and as a tool to evaluate and reflect on practice. Although the details of how any assessment of continued competence will be undertaken in the light of new legislation governing state registration have yet to be made explicit, developing a portfolio is unlikely to be a waste of time.

Different uses of portfolios

One of the purposes of this book is to show how portfolios may be used to present evidence of continuing professional development. However, portfolios have a variety of uses which all come under the umbrella of professional development. For example, portfolios may be used for demonstrating evidence of:

(1) Learning as a course participant
(2) Having achieved learning outcomes for assessment purposes
(3) Learning for academic accreditation
(4) Competence to practise
(5) Aptitude to support a job application
(6) Critical evaluation of practice
(7) Professional development and continuing competence
(8) Readiness for promotion
(9) Professional development as an educator
(10) Career development
(11) Skills and abilities that can be marketed

Learning as a course participant

Recognising that the technique of portfolio assessment was becoming better known and increasingly used in education, Brookfield (1995) advocated the use of the *participant learning portfolio*. The learner makes a record of experiences arising from a programme of study. This may involve analysing critical incidents, contributions to group discussions, written materials used to support the programme of study and personal learning experiences. The participant portfolio was said to allow the learner to become more reflective, to be able to recognise strengths and limitations more easily and to become more aware of the learning areas needing attention in the future. Feedback from the tutor could add value to the portfolio.

Showing achievement of learning outcomes for assessment purposes

Portfolios can be used as a mode of examination within an educational environment. A portfolio may be a method of presenting project work for examination or work compiled that shows evidence of meeting known assessment criteria. These are normally linked to the prescribed learning outcomes of the programme of study being undertaken. Learners should receive clear guidance about how to compile the portfolio and about the range (sufficiency and currency) of evidence that might be acceptable. The portfolio should always show evidence of reflection on both the contents and the nature of the learning experience (DfEE, 1998).

Learning for academic accreditation

Increasingly, higher education establishments are willing to recognise learning that has taken place outside of the academic environment, for example, in the workplace, and to give credit towards a course when it can be shown that this learning has taken place.

The learner is normally required to prepare and present evidence of when and how learning occurred, to show what learning outcomes were achieved and to indicate how new learning is to be used in the future. Certificates, project reports, personal reflective reports and testimonials can all contribute to the evidence that learning has taken place. These can be presented in a portfolio with a personal statement about what and how learning outcomes were achieved. The level, extent, relevance and currency of that learning will then be assessed by course staff to ascertain the amount of credit to be given towards meeting course requirements. Exemption from some aspect of the course of study may then be awarded.

Competence to practise

Some programmes leading to a professional qualification or to an award relating to practice, such as a National Vocational Qualification or a clinical practice teachers' course, are based on competencies. Evidence that these competencies have been achieved can be compiled and annotated in a portfolio.

Aptitude to support a job application

A portfolio can be compiled for a specific purpose and contain specially selected material that provides evidence of capability to do a job. The portfolio will contain evidence matched to each of the criteria listed on the job specification.

Critical evaluation of practice

In order to show continued competence in, and capability for, a job it may be necessary for an employee to show evidence that there has been ongoing evaluation of his or her practice. Evaluation can lead to improved performance in practice so evidence of this would be expected, and this can be presented in portfolio form. The portfolio might be a useful tool in a performance review and when formulating a personal development plan (PDP).

Professional development and continuing competence

A portfolio may be used to present evidence from a range of sources that competence has been maintained and improved and that skills have been developed to increasing levels of proficiency. For state registration purposes, the evidence must demonstrate continuing competence even though there may be evidence of enhanced competence or of the development of higher level skills and expertise. It may be compulsory or desirable for an employee to maintain a portfolio to demonstrate ongoing development between performance reviews. Reviews of performance will establish future goals to be achieved and the personal development plan for attaining them.

Readiness for promotion

Increasingly employers now specify performance criteria in the form of competencies or benchmarks that have to be achieved by employees seeking promotion.

In addition, a local pay agreement with a pay spine may require a particular level of competence to be achieved before an increment can be paid. Under the guidance of a mentor or coach, an employee can take steps to prepare for promotion by addressing these performance criteria. Details of additional competencies and how the criteria were met can be presented in a portfolio.

Professional development as an educator

A portfolio can be used to support any area of practice. It can show how learning and professional development are occurring and how these inform professional practice. For the majority of practitioners, a portfolio will show evidence of learning and professional development in the clinical field but Zubizarreta (1999) argued that a teaching portfolio kept by educators may also be a valuable tool to support reflective practice and promote improvement in teaching and learning. A teaching portfolio was defined by Zubizarreta as 'an evidence-based, written document in which a faculty member concisely organises selective details of teaching accomplishment and effort and uses such information to document his or her teaching enterprise' (1999, p. 52). He suggested that it could best be used for highlighting risks, challenges, disappointments and successes in the context of student learning. Maureen Shannon and Jonathan Rohrer (pers. comm.) saw the teaching portfolio as a means of scholarly documentation and personal reflection, leading to better planning for the future.

Career development

A portfolio developed for career purposes will need to show past achievement, current assets and future hopes and aspirations. The career portfolio is likely to be a personal collection of evidence of learning and expertise used to support job applications and career moves. An individual working in health or social care has a range of options for career development. He or she may opt for a career in:

- Clinical work, direct care or care management
- Service management
- Education
- Research
- Private practice and consultancy

A practitioner may choose any one area of work or any combination. He or she may progress from one area to another in the course of a career. A career portfolio will need to provide evidence of development and good practice with a focus on the chosen field of work. Each area can be sub-divided into categories. The portfolio may be used as evidence of good practice, as shown in the following sections.

Clinical work, direct care or care management

The portfolio may be used as evidence of good practice:

- In either specialist or general areas of practice
- With a specific user group
- In a particular practice location, e.g. primary care
- In the use of particular skills, techniques or equipment
- Using a well-developed knowledge base in a particular area
- By defining or developing the evidence base of practice
- Through publication of the evidence of good practice

Service management

The portfolio may indicate good practice in:

- Human resource management
- Staff supervision and development
- Service coordination and management
- Standard setting, audit and quality monitoring

- Project management
- Service development
- Budget monitoring or management
- Legal work
- Marketing and publicity

Education

The portfolio may be used to show evidence of good practice in:

- Understanding and application of the principles of learning and adult education
- Staff training, facilitation of learning and professional development
- The education of students
- Lecturing
- Mentoring, coaching or project supervision
- Course and curriculum development

Research

Again, good practice may be shown in:

- The development of research skills
- Searching and/or reviewing literature
- Critiquing research and related literature
- Particular research methodology
- Supporting research activity
- Initiating research projects
- Carrying out research
- Supervising research projects
- Disseminating research findings through reporting and publication
- Implementing research findings

Private work and consultancy

A portfolio may also be used as evidence for good practice in:

- Marketing and publicity
- Organisation and management
- Expertise in selected fields or skills of practice
- Medico-legal work
- Specialist clinics

The career development portfolio can show professional development over time. This can include evidence of educational and professional development and possibly the development of new personal attributes.

Skills and abilities that can be marketed

In view of the rapidly changing political and economic climate, Handy (1996) suggested that individuals can no longer expect jobs for life. It is now necessary to think differently about a career. A career can have many components. More people are becoming self-employed and combining jobs with private practice. Some people, who Handy refers to as portfolio people, develop a product, skill or service, assemble a portfolio that illustrates these assets and then market them. Given that many posts in the health and social care system, in education and in research are now offered as short, fixed-term contracts, there may be some merit in developing a portfolio for career purposes. The skills and abilities of the portfolio holder are clearly defined and can readily be reviewed by prospective employers.

Benefits of developing a portfolio

There is no doubt that portfolio development is a necessary but time-consuming activity that requires individuals to be disciplined, systematic and thorough in an approach to identifying, recording and presenting relevant evidence of learning and development. Although it takes time to select, record and order the information, the portfolio becomes the central location for all relevant information and this will undoubtedly save time and effort in the future (Lillyman & Evans, 1996).

Other benefits of developing a portfolio may be more long-term and not immediately obvious. They can be identified as:

(1)   Using portfolio development for self-development. The process of structuring, reflecting on and recording activity can be a significant learning process and can help to develop strategies for thinking, reasoning and communicating in professional practice.
(2)   Having a structured record and evidence of professional development over time to demonstrate ongoing competence to practise to meet legal and professional requirements whenever it is needed.
(3)   Having past achievements and future goals clearly defined.
(4)   Having clear goals and objectives with an action plan indicating how they might be fulfilled.
(5)   Having a range of material to hand from which can be selected relevant evidence to present as a personal profile for a particular purpose, for example, for educational, professional or career development purposes.

Cruickshank (1998) suggested that using a portfolio changes the way that learning is approached. It can make individuals more analytical and can facilitate the development of a positive approach to situations. While it may seem an onerous task, and might be construed as a lonely process, if it is tackled systematically in 'small chunks' it can become an integral part of professional practice with clear benefits to the owner.

Retrospective and prospective learning

Portfolio learning encompasses retrospective and prospective approaches. The retrospective approach essentially involves looking back at what has been done in order to identify and produce a record of past achievements, possibly with some commentary on the learning process. The prospective approach involves looking forward and entering into a process of planning, creating and pursuing learning opportunities. The process continues as learning opportunities occur. It is necessary to review what was learned and to explore how it should be applied in practice. Portfolio preparation requires a critical self-appraisal of current skills and knowledge levels. Reflection and careful analysis will allow areas of further development to be identified so that plans can be made for new learning. In this sense, portfolios offer individuals a unique opportunity to direct and monitor their own learning and development in support of their professional career (Bond, 1995).

Professional bodies and professional development

In respect of continuing professional development, professional bodies tend to see their prime responsibility as the promotion, monitoring and evaluation of professional standards so that the public can be assured of the competence of the membership. Secondly, professional bodies provide support to the membership in relation to professional activity and development. They serve as a resource, providing guidance on continuing professional development and information to support CPD activity. Most professionals would see CPD activity as a partnership responsibility between the employee, employer, education provider and professional body. Professional bodies tend to provide the benchmark against which competent performance might be assessed, and most have schemes that support post-qualifying education, training and professional development to enable the membership to maintain professional skills, widen knowledge and develop high levels of competence.

Summary

There are a number of different uses for portfolios. In essence, they are all concerned with demonstrating the achievements and capabilities of their owners. The one thing to be said, however, is that they are all going to be presented differently in ways that reflect the interests, priorities and intentions of those individuals who have compiled them. The next chapter explores ways of selecting and presenting relevant material in portfolio form.

References

Alsop, A. (1995) The professional portfolio – purpose, process and practice. Part 1: portfolios and professional practice. *British Journal of Occupational Therapy* **58** (7), 299–302.

Bond, C. (1995) A portfolio-based approach to professional development. In *Continuing Professional Development – Perspectives on CPD in Practice* (S. Clyne, ed.). Kogan Page, London.

Brookfield, S. (1995) *Becoming a Critically Reflective Teacher*. Jossey-Bass, San Francisco.

Brown, R.A. (1992) *Portfolio Development and Profiling for Nurses*. Quay Publications, Lancaster.

Brown, S. & Knight, P. (1994) *Assessing Learners in Higher Education*. Kogan Page, London.

Calman, K.C. (1998) A Review of Continuing Professional Development in General Practice. Report by the Chief Medical Officer, Department of Health, London.

Cannon, T. (1992) *Basic Marketing – Principles and Practice*, 3rd edn. Cassell, London.

Chartered Society of Physiotherapy (1994) *The Professional Development Diary*. Information Paper CPD5. CSP, London.

College of Occupational Therapists (1994) *Post-qualifying Guidance and Directory*. College of Occupational Therapists, London.

Cruickshank, L. (1998) Professional Development Programme: College of Occupational Therapists' Portfolio Part 1. Occupational Therapy News, College of Occupational Therapists, London.

DfEE (1998) *A Common Framework for Learning*. Department for Education and Employment, UK.

Handy, C. (1996) *Beyond Certainty*. Arrow Books, London.

Hull, C. & Redfern, L. (1996) *Profiles and Portfolios: A Guide for Nurses and Midwives*. Macmillan Press, Basingstoke.

Lillyman, S. & Evans, B. (1996) *Designing a Personal Portfolio/Profile – A Workbook for Healthcare Professionals*. Quay Books, Salisbury.

Redman, W. (1994) *Portfolios for Development: A Guide for Trainers and Managers*. Kogan Page, London.

Zubizarreta, J. (1999) Teaching portfolios: an effective strategy for faculty development in occupational therapy. *American Journal of Occupational Therapy* **53** (1), 51–5.

Chapter 3
Developing a Portfolio

Getting started

The one thing to be said about putting together a portfolio is the sooner you get started the better. It ought not to be necessary to wait until it is a requirement to have evidence of continued competence. CPD should be seen as a voluntary activity, as a professional responsibility and as a process for maintaining competence in practice. Take the initiative yourself and, if you have not already done so, start your portfolio now. But where do you start?

Putting together a portfolio is not nearly as daunting as it sounds. It is a relatively straightforward activity, if a little time consuming, especially at first, and it need not be expensive. There is no need, unless you want to, to invest in a professionally produced CPD package. You can compile and present the material yourself in your own way. If you do want to use a commercially produced portfolio you will be prompted to think about yourself, your achievements and other professional activity in a structured way, but it is not essential to use one, and you can achieve the same result without the expense. There are various options for presenting the material in portfolio form which will be addressed later. The first thing is to think about what needs to be in the portfolio and to make a start at putting it together.

Cruickshank (1998) suggested that you start with the factual aspects of your career that can be recorded in a fairly straightforward way. These might be perceived as being easier to complete than some of the more evaluative aspects of the portfolio or those where you need to think carefully about plans for the future. All of these will need to be addressed at some stage, but putting together the factual aspects will get you started. If the thought of putting a portfolio together does seem an overwhelming task then it is best to start in a small way and develop the portfolio at a pace that you can manage. The overall framework can emerge over time.

Completing the process of portfolio development involves assembling material under three headings that represent your past, present and future professional activity. They are addressed here in turn but it does not matter in which order you tackle them. It is wise to start where you feel most confident.

Past activity

Your CV

One good place to start is with what you can readily recall about your career to date. You may already have a curriculum vitae (CV) that shows your qualifications and career moves. If you do not have a CV then now is the time to prepare one.

Start by making several lists that reflect your professional activity and your career from the point when you qualified as a health professional (or before if relevant) to the present time. You should list, with relevant dates:

- Your formal qualifications
- Your employment record
- Details of the professional roles and responsibilities you have held
- Other professional activities in which you have participated
- Other courses that you have undertaken

This will not necessarily demonstrate your professional development but will at least serve as a point of reference and a foundation on which to build your portfolio. The details will eventually be compiled into a CV but as Cruickshank (1998) pointed out, a CV is only a list of accomplishments over time. A portfolio needs to provide a fuller picture of the process and outcomes of professional activities undertaken. In time, you will need to expand on some of the roles and responsibilities you have had and to summarise the key experiences and learning achieved in each of the roles.

The next thing to do is to locate and bring together any evidence of:

- Your qualifications (certificates, awards)
- The courses that you have done (programmes of events, statements of attendance)
- The roles and responsibilities you have had (testimonials, job descriptions, reports, notes from meetings)

Any documentation that verifies past professional activity can be useful. All of it, or a carefully selected part of it, can eventually be assembled and catalogued in some meaningful way. It is an idea to take photocopies of certificates in order to preserve the original.

If recently qualified, you might wish to show your activities both before and after qualification. Include details of clinical placements or fieldwork education and any special experiences that helped you to learn and to develop professionally prior to qualification. Did you have any challenging or out-of-the-ordinary placements or learning opportunities during your course? Did you hold any particular role or have responsibility such as course representative or committee member?

Now you should bring this material together in a CV. Some of the headings you might use are shown in Table 3.1. Make sure that you date your CV and update it regularly. If you wish to use it when applying for a new job or for promotion you have the information to hand. You can then select relevant information to present a succinct CV specifically related to the position for which you are applying.

Table 3.1 General headings for a Curriculum Vitae

1 Personal details Name Address Telephone number E-mail address
2 Present employment Job title Place of employment Telephone number Name of employer Address of employer

3 Professional and academic qualifications

Date of award	Title of award	Awarding body

4 Record of employment

Date of appointment	Post held	Name and address
Date of leaving	Key responsibilities	of employer

5 Summary of professional activities

From/	Professional activity
To (*date*)	e.g. professional roles held
	projects undertaken
	publications
	papers/posters presented
	teaching experiences
	events organised
	research activity

Another way of presenting details of your career is to summarise activity in each post previously held. Fig. 3.1 provides a model for this. Dates of employment, key functions, professional roles and activities undertaken while in the post can be highlighted. A series of these could show your professional development over time Questions that you might ask yourself particularly about your most recent professional experiences are as follows:

(1)   What key responsibilities have you had that have enhanced your understanding of practice?

From: (date)   **To:** (date) **Post held:** **Key functions:**   **Professional roles:**   **Professional activities:**   **Professional achievements:**   **Professional education and qualifications gained:**   **Projects/publications/research completed:**

Fig. 3.1   Summary of post held and professional activity and achievements.

(2)   What new skills have you learnt, how did you learn them and how are you applying them in practice?

(3)   Which skills have you developed to a more advanced level and how are they being used in your work?

(4)   What new areas or fields of practice have you visited or worked in and how have these added to your knowledge and expertise?

(5)   What significant books or articles have you read that have helped you to update or upgrade your knowledge or practice?

(6)   What other experiences have you had from which you learned something? These may be formal, informal or chance experiences.

(7)   What courses have you undertaken and how has your practice, or your approach to practice, developed or changed as a result?

These questions may help you to reflect particularly on how you have developed in the last six to twelve months. Note that the answers to some of the questions may emerge from many more experiences than just conferences, courses or study days you have attended. Different people, places and events may all have made an impact in some way or another and you should record anything that is noteworthy. The way in which you have applied new knowledge in practice should be emphasised.

Professional activity and achievements

It is usual to think quite widely about professional activity and achievements. Professional activity covers a broad range of experiences and tasks that you do in addition to the primary responsibilities of your job. Some of the questions you might ask yourself are:

(1) Have you undertaken or contributed to any special projects or been a member of a working party?
(2) Have you been involved in any committee as a member, for example:
   - within or representing your service?
   - for your professional body?
   - representing a special interest group or area of practice?
(3) Have you organised or coordinated any special event, for example, a careers evening, open day, study day or conference?
(4) Have you 'acted up' within your service or taken on extra responsibilities on a temporary basis?
(5) Have you given any talks on your field of practice or your service?
(6) Have you undertaken any teaching – provided clinical education, in-service education or given lectures?
(7) Have you contributed to or undertaken any research?
(8) Have you written any leaflets or information sheets for service users?
(9) Have you reviewed, audited or developed any part of your service?
(10) Have you introduced new working methods or written protocols, policies or procedures?
(11) Have you published any articles or books?
(12) Have you presented any papers or posters at a conference?

Again, this is not a definitive list but it may prompt you to think about the range of activity in which you might have engaged and from which you might have learned. You can either make a definitive list, giving dates and summarising the responsibilities involved, or you can list them under each post held. You will need to bring together any evidence of your activity. Where activities are extensive, for example in research, education or publication, you might set aside a special section in your portfolio. If you have volumes of evidence you may need to be selective in favour of more recent activities, provided they are relevant, or to focus more exclusively on a particular theme related to your practice.

Professional education and qualifications

Educational activity might include workshops, professional visits, in-service or external courses or conferences that you have attended. For as many of them as you can, note the dates, list the key points that you learned from them and indicate how this learning has influenced, or will influence, your practice. If you still have the programme available then this will support your evidence of learning. Make a particular note of any new insights, thoughts or ideas and any changes in your approach to practice that the educational activity has prompted.

Specialist skills and expertise

Over time you may have developed some of your skills and expertise to quite a sophisticated level. Through regular exposure to, participation in, and exploration of the subject area you may have gained proficiency in a selected aspect of your practice. Other practitioners may consult you and use your experience because you have built up expertise over a period of time. One of the things that you might therefore do for your portfolio is to make explicit how this expertise has developed because it is clearly something that you and other people value and it is relevant to practice.

Sometimes expertise develops by default. For example, because no-one else was there, you stepped in to do the job and somehow this aspect of the job has now become your domain. Sometimes expertise develops because of outside interests beyond the job. You bring these interests to the job and allow them to influence the way that you work. For example, an occupational therapist who enjoys gardening at home may select this activity as a medium for intervention.

You may take a particular approach or opt for a particular intervention strategy because you can draw on expertise over and above that gained in your initial qualifying professional education. A practitioner may be able to use their additional qualifications and interests to complement their professional skills. Sometimes expertise develops through practice because, by showing an interest in a particular facet of practice, expertise has built up incrementally. As a therapist, you may have sought employment in positions that have allowed you to exploit and develop that area of expertise. Expertise may relate to skills developed in a defined area of clinical practice with service users but it might also relate to an aspect of management, education, research, supervision, mentorship or any one of a range of activities that contribute to service provision. It is important that you think widely about the expertise that you might have, and not just about the skills you use in direct contact with service users.

It is important that your skills and expertise are identified in the portfolio and the ways in which they have been developed are made explicit. Your participation in courses, your reading around the subject matter and your engagement in practice and/or research may be indicators of your professional development.

Other significant experiences

Another way of generating thoughts and ideas about what to record in a portfolio is to start by making a list of past experiences that have been particularly meaningful for you. They do not necessarily have to be work-related, they could be life experiences, but they will be quite vivid in your memory because they were significant to you in some way. In each case summarise what happened and the effect that it had on you. From the summary you should be able to extract some points that you learned or that are going to act as triggers for future reference. List these points as a reminder of what you discovered from the experience. The learning points may relate to:

- Things that you know now that you did not know before
- Things that you can do now that you could not do before
- Steps that you now know that you need to take to avoid a problem or to ensure a satisfactory outcome
- Insights that you had about a situation
- Things that you have learned about yourself
- Attributes you have developed
- Links or relationships you have discovered between different phenomena
- Consequences of taking a particular course of action that you had not realised or foreseen
- Effects that a course of action had on other people
- The most appropriate sequence of events discovered after trial and error

It may be possible to summarise two or three experiences, linked or unrelated, from which a common set of learning points emerges. Practice in examining your own experiences will be valuable when it comes to exploring critical incidents involving other people. Logging recent and future experiences, for example those shown in Fig. 3.2, may help you build up a picture of how you have developed over time.

Current activity

Keeping a diary or log

Starting in a small way to develop your portfolio can just mean noting on a regular basis significant events and what you have learned from them (Fig. 3.2). Keep a log of the things that you discover that you did not know before. To start with, this may be no more than a record of meaningful events and snippets of learning, but at least it is a start. A more sophisticated learning log would comprise a description of each significant event from which learning occurred and an analysis and personal interpretation of the situation in respect of your own practice.

Role analysis

A more structured activity that can contribute to the development of your portfolio and, for that matter, to your career development, is *role analysis*. The way to do this is first to list all the roles in which you currently engage within

Date	Professional activity or learning experience	Key learning points	Application to practice

Fig 3.2 Log of professional activity.

your employment or work life. You should also include any other roles that align with your employment but are not part of it, for example voluntary work. Possible work-related roles might include:

- Clinician/practitioner
- Teacher
- Educator
- Coach
- Consultant
- Representative
- Supervisor
- Mentor

- Manager
- Project worker
- Researcher
- Committee member
- Steward
- Keyworker
- Care manager
- Lecturer/practitioner

This is not a definitive list and you may think of different roles. There are probably far more than you first think. There may also be others, such as advisor, counsellor or volunteer that you engage in outside work but that clearly complement your work activity.

The next thing to do is to identify what all these roles entail. You can then go on to ask yourself other questions such as:

- What expectations are there of me in this role? (Different people, including yourself, may have different expectations).
- What knowledge, skills or competence do I need to fulfil each role?
- Am I judged to be competent, proficient or expert in each role? This may be different for each role.
- What knowledge, skills or competence do I still need to develop in order to fulfil the role to expectations?

Of course, it may turn out to be worrying if you realise that you are trying to do the job without the necessary skills or competence in the roles that you have. Perhaps you have taken the job early in your career or taken over someone else's responsibilities in their absence or because someone has left the service. You may have still to develop the skills needed for some aspects of the role. At least by recognising this you can start to do something about it.

Finally, for every role that you have identified, write down what professional development activity you have undertaken in the last one to two years in support of that role. What have you learned or what have you done towards developing yourself in each of the roles you have listed? You should try to translate the development activity into learning outcomes to show what has been achieved (see Chapter 10). You should then be able to summarise how the learning activity has been or will be put into practice. In this way you ought to be able to show that learning has taken place and how it is being used or will be used to modify or develop your practice in the future. If you wanted to, you could prepare a fairly detailed, reflective account of your role development over a period of time to add to your portfolio. Additionally, you could ask colleagues or other significant people to provide a testimonial for you in relation to a role that you have undertaken. This would provide a different kind of evidence in support of what you have said.

You can tabulate the information about roles and date it. If you have been thorough and examined each role in turn, you should be able to see where the gaps are in your professional development. If there are roles that you are undertaking but for which you have not identified any development activity, the gaps on your list may indicate some of your future development needs. These gaps in your knowledge, skills and competence can be translated into an action plan that details the way in which you intend to develop the skills you need or to enhance the skills you need to a different, and perhaps more appropriate, level. Fig. 3.3 shows how this might look. The role analysis, action plan and learning that ensues should also be documented for the portfolio.

Current role	Recent development activity to support the role	Future development needs

Fig.3.3 Role analysis and development needs.

Situation analysis

You may hold many roles within your employment and asking some of the questions above should have identified many of your strengths and limitations. As part of the exploration of your current situation it is worth asking some further questions about your employment so that a picture emerges of where you are now and where you might wish to be. For example:

(1) Are you in a job that you enjoy? If not what are your plans?
(2) Is the job linked to your longer term career goals? What comes next?
(3) What are the key responsibilities of the job?
(4) Are you sufficiently skilled to be able to undertake all aspects of the job competently? If not where are the gaps and what are the deficits?
(5) Is the job evolving whereby you need to be thinking about developing new skills or more advanced skills?
(6) Are you likely to move into a new practice environment where you will be expected to use existing skills in a new context?
(7) Are you expecting to change your job soon and what will that mean for skill development?

Future activity and goals

Bond (1995) made it clear that, like any car journey on which you might embark, you do not set out without having some idea about where you are going or want to get to, and the same needs to be said about portfolio development. Defined goals should indicate the place you need to be and should give direction. They will help you to choose the most appropriate pace and route to get you there. Learning will be a part of the process and the pace of learning may be at an accelerated rate or via a slower route. Learning opportunities will be chosen accordingly and any deviation from the chosen course will be carefully considered for its merits.

Career analysis

A performance review and your personal development plans will establish short term needs and goals but periodically you will need to review your total career to date and to create a vision of your career for the future. Your long-term goals and needs should be identified and set out as longer term plans. The questions above about your current situation may help you to consider where you are now but you may need to ask yourself further questions about your future aims, for example:

(1) Are you aiming to stay in the same area of practice throughout your career?
(2) Are you intending to remain with the same employer?

(3)   Do you have aspirations for developing your present role and for enhancing your expertise in your current specialty?

(4)   Do you want to take on additional roles and responsibilities in your job, for example, clinical supervisor, manager, educator or researcher?

(5)   Do you want to add additional experiences to your work, for example by exploring the evidence base for your practice?

(6)   Do you have any aspiration to move into professional or general management, into education, private practice or consultancy?

(7)   Are you anticipating a break in service and having to make plans for maintaining competence?

Can you visualise the sort of work that you might aim to be doing in five years time? This may seem like a long time away and difficult to predict. It may also be difficult to predict what service provision might look like in that time and what effect any future organisational change will have, but it is still important to have longer term personal aims and goals to work towards in your career. A strategy for achieving these goals can then be developed to give direction even if it needs to be revised because of changing circumstances.

Some of the ways in which you might identify future plans and goals have already been noted. You might have a continuing development plan to enhance your knowledge, skills and expertise in a particular area of practice, or a personal development plan from your performance review. Apart from meeting service needs, however, it is important that you set your own agenda and identify your personal goals for future career development.

Personal plans

Any plans that you have, both now and in the future, may be influenced by personal and family commitments or other personal plans. Plans for future professional activity will need to be realistic and to take account of any known plans or circumstances relating to your private life. There is only so much that you can cope with at any one time so both your personal and professional activities need to be considered together.

Presenting the evidence

It is important that the time you spend developing your portfolio is productive time, so you do need to decide on a strategy and format for the presentation of material. This will help you to concentrate your efforts on selected aspects of your career and professional development rather than randomly present a collection of material in a haphazard way that has no internal consistency. You may choose to work through in chronological order or to use themes. As long as the portfolio is comprehensive and well-ordered, with clearly defined sections, cross referenced where necessary, and with an index, it does not matter how it is compiled.

Hull & Redfern (1996) offer some practical advice on the organisation of a portfolio in that they remind us that someone else may need to make sense of your portfolio (or of selected parts of it) and not just you. It is possible that the person reading or assessing your portfolio may not know you so it is important that the information in the portfolio is accessible, clear to read and easy to follow so that it makes sense. It is also worth remembering that it is your learning from experience that is important and not just your experience.

Obviously, if you are presenting a portfolio that has to meet given criteria then the selection and presentation of the most appropriate evidence is crucial. Criteria are relevant if you are presenting material for formal examination. Equally they will be relevant if statutory criteria or guidelines come into force for the assessment of continued competence to practise.

Again, it is worth remembering that you are not trying to tell everything that you know because the portfolio would be too unwieldy. As Hull & Redfern (1996) remarked, the best presentation is often the one that is concise and related directly to what is being assessed. If you cannot be selective in what you present then the reader might assume that you do not know what is relevant and what is not, and so cannot make judgements. Irrelevant material may lose you credibility.

Ownership

The main thing to remember when putting your portfolio together is that it is *your portfolio*. You have total ownership of it and you can present as little or as much information as you like, in any way that you like. You are collecting the evidence of your continuing professional development and so have a free rein when it comes to decisions about presentation. If you ever have to present a portfolio to someone else's specifications, for example, for accreditation or assessment for a defined purpose, then you can extract relevant material from your own portfolio just for that purpose and arrange it in accordance with the specification.

If your employer requires you to maintain a portfolio, either manually or as part of a department computerised system, you should expect to see and agree a policy and procedure for accessing, sharing and retaining information contained in the portfolio. Confusion can easily arise if the expectations of your employer are different to your expectations about who has access to your portfolio and for what it might be used. It may be that a manager has purchased portfolio hardware or software for you but this does not automatically give him or her the right to access your portfolio's contents. If you are required to keep records in portfolio form at work you should know at least:

- Whether it supports a system of performance review, and how?
- Where records will be kept?

- Who will have access to them and for what purpose?
- Who can update the records?
- What happens to the records when you leave?

You may choose only to keep essential information about your CPD at work and to keep your main portfolio at home.

Portfolio – public or private?

Essentially the portfolio is a private document but if it is to serve its purpose as evidence of continuing professional development then some of it at least will need to be made public. It is essential that you consider whether all or only some of your portfolio is to be open to public scrutiny and then present the material accordingly. It is possible to have a two-part portfolio where one side is public and the other is kept very private. This provides choice about the presentation of the material. Obviously, material that is in any way confidential needs to be maintained as confidential in the private side. Another range of material may need to be treated as sensitive and not necessarily made widely available to any reader. If you keep a professional reflective diary or log and it forms part of the portfolio, you will probably wish to keep this aspect confidential and only provide a summary of the interpretation of the material for public use. Material that is collated and presented in an orderly fashion can quickly provide the foundations from which you can extract a smaller collection of material on a given topic for a given purpose.

If you work with a mentor you must decide how much of your portfolio to share. It is not unreasonable for you to agree with a mentor a code of confidentiality that you can both respect regarding what is seen, discussed and ultimately presented. If you must present a portfolio to your manager to demonstrate your professional development and how your plans are taking shape, then it is essential to have a departmental policy in place.

Confidentiality

Some of the evidence of your CPD, especially if it has come from a service, may be judged to be confidential. Documents such as minutes from meetings and unpublished reports may not be taken from the service for private use. Clearly there may be limits to what can reasonably be included in the portfolio and the confidentiality of services and service users has to be respected at all times. Nothing should be held on file that can be directly attributed to a service or to an individual service user unless you have explicit permission to use it for your portfolio.

Early decisions

There are some early decisions to be made about the presentation of the material in portfolio form. The first two key decisions are:

(1)   Do you want to buy an 'off-the-peg' tool that offers you the structure within which to record your activities, or do you want to create the structure of your portfolio yourself so that you can shape it according to your own needs and interests?
(2)   Do you want to use a computerised or manual system?

Creating your own portfolio or using one 'off-the-peg'?

Basically, an off-the-peg design, in either a manual version or as software, creates the structure in which you build your portfolio. A number of designs are on the market. Some professional bodies have had portfolio packages specially designed to meet their members' needs and they can be purchased in either manual form or as computer software. There is an initial financial outlay and the choice depends on personal preference but will often be influenced by an individual's confidence in using information technology and his or her access to resources. These prepared packages can be helpful to get you started quickly and efficiently and they can promote the thorough and systematic presentation of a large range of material in portfolio form.

It must be stressed, however, that a system that pre-defines the structure and format of a portfolio is not at all necessary. It might even be considered a hindrance and an unnecessary expense. A pre-defined structure may not suit the way in which you want to work. The sections may not be ordered or categorised in the way you would wish. If this is the case then you might be well advised to consider creating your own version, personalised for your own use.

A portfolio can be built up from scratch, for example, by using a large, good quality lever arch file, polythene pockets and some card dividers. It is important to work systematically and to create sections to hold the material you present and to index it and cross reference it carefully in order to locate the material efficiently.

Using software

Increasingly information technology is being used to support CPD activity. Packages such as the Professional Development Programme offered by the College of Radiographers and College of Occupational Therapists can be purchased by members to be installed on their computers at home.

The software is intended to help individuals manage and keep a record of their CPD activity. Packages come with a helpful user guide. The software is struc-

tured to ask users a number of pertinent questions relating to work and professional experience. Achievements and capabilities are explored and answers
can be logged into the system. There is guidance on how to form personal
objectives for the short and longterm, taking into consideration the user's preferred career direction. There is a capacity to update the records and review
achievements against stated objectives. The CPD record and development plan
can always be up-to-date and ready for use whenever required.

Manual systems

If you prefer to use a manual system but still like a structure to prompt you to
identify activities and achievements, several commercial manual portfolios are
on the market. The packages made available as software tend also to be available
in manual form. Alternatively you can buy a portfolio file with sections already

Table 3.2 Possible section headings for a portfolio.

Index
Any flow-charts as a guide to using the portfolio

Personal details
Name, address, telephone number, e-mail address
State registration number
Professional association membership number
CV
References, testimonials
Overview of career

PAST ACTIVITY

Professional qualifications
Academic qualifications
Additional accredited education

Professional education
Courses, conferences, workshops attended }   details of associated learning
Non-traditional education activity   }   and application to practice

Professional employment
Details of posts held, key responsibilities, achievements
Details of additional professional roles, responsibilities and achievements

Professional activity
Membership of professional committees, working groups
Projects completed
Teaching and lecturing activities
Events organised
Publications
Conference papers or posters presented
Research activity

labelled and a guide to help you to present evidence of your own CPD. It is worth checking the labels before buying the portfolio because portfolios are available for a wide variety of professions and sections may not always be appropriate. There is no real difference between the manual and software systems that have been tailor-made to a profession's needs and specifications, and it comes down to personal preference. Manual systems are arguably more portable and visual, although if completed with hand-written entries they may not be as smartly presented as material produced by software programmes.

Creating your own portfolio

It is not difficult and it is perfectly acceptable to compile a portfolio to your own specifications. Normally it is useful to present material in an A4 ring binder, perhaps making good use of transparent polythene pockets to hold papers of

Table 3.2 *Contd.*

Specialist skills and expertise Evidence of development of specialist skills and expertise **Other significant experiences** Personal reflections on selected experiences **Evidence of recent professional updating** Critical incident reviews, case studies, audit activity Abstracts of research/projects/papers/posters Reviews of books/articles read Reflections on visits, secondments, discussions or other experiences Personal reflections on personal and professional development Plans/photographs/videos that depict progress of projects and projects completed **CURRENT ACTIVITY** **Roles analysis** Role analysis and development needs **Personal development plan** Summary of performance review and review of previous objectives and learning Short term personal and professional goals Current professional objectives Personal development plan Details of any learning contracts in place **Current projects** Details of any current projects, learning activity, research or other commitments **FUTURE ACTIVITY** Future aspirations and career direction Longer term objectives, personal and professional goals

irregular sizes. Many types of quite sophisticated files and binders are now on the market so there is plenty of choice. However, as a start, a file for a portfolio does not have to be expensive to be useful and presentable.

The portfolio really needs to be structured in sections. The headings shown in Table 3.2 may help you present material systematically but if these headings do not meet your needs then create your own. Remember your portfolio is yours and no one else will have access to it without your permission so whatever system you use only has to be acceptable to you.

Documentation

Documentation to support and verify the activities you have undertaken is important. This may be as straightforward as certificates of qualifications, courses attended, awards or achievements. Other documents might include programmes of study days, workshops, conferences, abstracts of papers presented or copies of papers given at conferences. A journal review of a paper you presented, feedback sheets on presentations made or reports that you have written could all provide evidence. Other evidence might include:

- Copies of reports, documents, information leaflets
- Published articles
- Abstracts of papers or posters presented
- Curricula of courses designed
- Protocols/policy documents
- Abstracts
- Critical incident reviews
- Critical reviews of literature
- Review of learning contract
- Case studies/stories
- Videos
- Photographs/drawings/plans
- References/testimonials/letters
- Published reviews of your work by others

A separate container will need to accommodate the evidence of CPD particularly if you are recording activity using a computer. Chapter 10 further examines evidence of learning and provides some other examples of types of evidence.

Qualities of a portfolio

The key qualities of a portfolio are that it should be clear and comprehensive but concise. It is essential to be selective in what is recorded and held as part of the portfolio. You do not need everything, but if the main purpose of the portfolio is to show professional development then anything that is included has to contribute to meeting that goal. If it is limited to continuing professional development then it is worth bearing in mind the purpose of CPD, once again summarised below:

- To develop personal qualities
- To enhance professional and technical skills
- To maintain, enhance and broaden professional knowledge
- To maintain quality and relevance of professional services
- To develop and enhance practice
- To prepare for changing roles in service delivery

The contents of a portfolio relating to CPD should therefore be presented in such a way as to show evidence of achieving its purpose. It is also important for the portfolio to be reflective and to show evidence of self-evaluation and critical awareness. It needs to show evidence of learning, of updating professional knowledge and to demonstrate professional growth.

Table 3.3 provides a checklist that might help you shape your portfolio, help inform your decisions about what should be included (or left out) and help you to locate the material quickly.

Table 3.3 Checklist for a portfolio.

Does your portfolio:
• Present evidence carefully selected according to the purpose of the portfolio?
• Present evidence in a structured way?
• Show how evidence is to be interpreted in the light of any assessment criteria?
• Set the evidence in the context of your personal goals?
• Present information that is well-ordered, indexed and cross-referenced so that information can be found quickly and easily by other readers?
• Present material concisely, comprehensively, clearly and neatly?
• Demonstrate reflection, analysis, critical awareness, self evaluation?
• Indicate learning outcomes from various experiences?
• Show how learning and new knowledge are being or will be applied in practice?
• Indicate plans and the direction of future development activity?

It is important to view a portfolio as a positive record of personal strengths and achievements and as a proactive approach to keeping up to date and to developing skills and competence. It may be an approach to continual learning but it should not just be a facility for identifying gaps and limitations and the way in which they will be addressed. A portfolio should be a celebration of attainment that is an honest and meaningful account of your personal learning and professional development.

References

Bond, C. (1995) A portfolio-based approach to professional development. In *Continuing Professional Development – Perspectives on CPD in Practice* (S. Clyne, ed.). Kogan Page, London.

Cruickshank, L. (1998) Professional Development Programme: College of Occupational Therapists' Portfolio Part 1. Occupational Therapy News, College of Occupational Therapists, London

Hull, C. & Redfern, L. (1996) *Profiles and Portfolios – A Guide for Nurses and Midwives.* Macmillan, Basingstoke.

Chapter 4
Building a Career

A personal career

Creating a portfolio by recalling your past professional activity and logging it is all very well, but your continuing professional development really means taking a longer term view of your plans for the future. Career goals need to be formed, however loosely, so that you can build your career and direct your learning and professional activity accordingly. When you have some vision about the likely direction of your career and possible career moves, your learning for personal, professional and career development can be integrated into one development plan. Once upon a time a career meant pursuing a profession or occupation for life, but we now know that this is no longer the norm. A career has now come to represent a series of steps in employment that may be related by some theme or purpose, or that reflect different employment challenges. One positive aspect of employment in the new climate is that it is becoming easier, as well as increasingly common, to change direction within a career or to change a career path altogether. Some of you may already have had another career before entering a health care profession. You may even be drawing on the experiences from your former employment in your current job.

Jobs for life no longer exist and opportunities for career progression within flattened organisational structures are often difficult to find. However, on the brighter side, there is now more scope when making career plans and choices to follow a varied course in employment. Within the health and social care sectors there is room for movement between jobs, roles and organisations. Skills acquired in professional education can be used in many different ways and transferred to new situations. Mobility is now an accepted aspect of a career path. Taking breaks from employment to pursue personal projects and interests is now also an accepted part of professional life. It is always possible to return to health care after a break in service, provided that steps are taken to maintain competence. As an alternative to climbing the career ladder and taking on more responsibility it is also common to look for sideways moves in order to gain different kinds of experience and fulfil personal aspirations and career goals. A map of one professional's career will therefore be very different from another's.

A career step is another stage of your journey through professional life that may at some time have been (and may still be) guided by a vision of how you choose and expect to use your time in employment. Moves may be planned in advance or may come about as opportunities arise. Where there is a clear vision of where you want to be, then development plans can be formulated. In order to take advantage of career opportunities you will need to know where your strengths are and of any gaps in your knowledge that need to be filled. This is essential for seeking future employment. In new situations your employer will need to recognise your limitations and help you to make plans for developing those skills that are essential to the job you are doing. So in any new job there is likely to be new learning and even as a well qualified and experienced professional, your learning will be ongoing.

A learning professional

Those of you who are qualified and registered as a member of one of the professions allied to medicine will have been through a course of professional education approved under the Professions Supplementary to Medicine Act 1960. Your competence to practise will have been demonstrated and the professional qualification awarded, giving you a licence to practise. With your qualification, however, come all the responsibilities expected of a professional, including respect for the ethical principles of causing no harm and doing the best for each service user and the expectation that you will continue to develop your knowledge and skills and use them to serve the best interests of the public.

'Qualification is a *rite of passage*', a 'landmark in the process of professional socialisation' (Eraut, 1994, p. 159). It is a time when learning is validated and translated into a licence to practise as a member of a profession. The qualification serves both as a sign of personal achievement and as evidence that a milestone has been reached in the progress of lifelong learning (Longworth & Davies, 1996). However, as Eraut also pointed out, qualification may signify 'a critical change in the status of a professional and mark a decline in the amount of time formally allocated to professional learning' (1994, p. 217). The suggestion here is that as soon as education is no longer formally structured, practitioners may not set aside time for learning with the same degree of commitment. It is easy to think of the point of qualification as being the ultimate achievement of a personal goal that has already made huge demands in terms of your time and effort. Personal sacrifices may have been considerable in the commitment to gaining the qualification, and the last thing that most qualifying practitioners are likely to want in the immediate future is to engage in continuing professional development. Yet this is the commitment that each qualifying practitioner is implicitly making as he or she accepts the role and responsibilities of a professional. Eraut (1994) advised us that the point of qualification should not trigger a break in the learning process. Qualification should not be the end point but the start of professional development that will be ongoing. Continuity of learning is a crucial factor in both the consolidation of your learning and in your professional growth.

One of the points to be made in this book is that competence may only be short-lived unless continuing professional development does take place. A number of authors have noted that knowledge is time-limited. Clyne (1995), for example, stated that it is no longer possible for professionals to practise the same things in the same way for the whole of their working life. Even though Eraut (1994, p. 11) acknowledged that learning continues well beyond initial qualification, he also argued that good professional practice decays over time (p. 40). Ashton (1992) commented that professional knowledge can be out of date in less than five years. Haines (1997) weighed up the evidence for the limited life of competence and professional knowledge. Obsolescence of knowledge was put at between two and five years before it was superseded. She concluded that professional competency is a perishable commodity and that the acquisition of initial registration qualifications is only the first step towards continuous learning. Thus there is a need for ongoing learning just to remain competent, regardless of the need to develop and improve competence. Given the pace of change in professional work (Downs, 1993) where increasingly complex and specialised work requires constant updating (Clyne, 1995), the real life of competence may be much reduced. In order to remain competent to practise, learning must be ongoing, especially as competence has been described as being context-specific (Hollis, 1997) and the practice environment constantly changes. Education and training must therefore become a continuous lifelong process to keep abreast of change (Clyne, 1995).

A learning professional thus has two areas of responsibility, one professional and one personal. The first is to keep up to date with the changing nature of practice so as to be able to continue to practise safely and competently, taking account of environmental changes. The second is to plan and engage in learning activity that is going to support career intentions and personal development plans. Both require insight into different learning strategies that can support professional development.

In sum, the educational programme leading to a professional qualification is only the start of a learning process that, at a point in time, assures the public that a practitioner is competent to practise. All too often, however, the point of qualification is seen as the point at which formal learning should cease instead of a point on the continuum of lifelong learning that keeps the practising professional abreast of changes and able to demonstrate both personal and professional effectiveness and growth. While keeping up-to-date is a professional responsibility, each professional has a responsibility to map out potential career moves and to ensure that development activities are planned to support them.

The professional journey

The professional career is a journey through which each professional travels at his or her own pace and in a direction that is largely self-determined. Much of the preparation for this journey takes place through a pre-registration qualifying programme in an educational environment, as has already been said, but the real journey begins at the point of qualification. A professional career is therefore not just a journey but a 'learning career'.

The educational programme leading to professional qualification is a journey in itself. It is well planned, has particular highlights, takes different directions and involves learning about new cultures and ways of doing things. Learners' experiences are explored for new meaning and understanding and stored as memories in some useful way for future reference. In many ways, professional education is like a package tour where the journey is set in a pre-defined framework. Optional visits and experiences are interspersed with necessary elements. Each member of the group will have different interests and gain different insights and benefits from the experiences. The main feature of the tour is that there is access to a guide (a lecturer) to help steer the journey and to act as a resource to enable each group member to appreciate and interpret the experiences in a personally meaningful way. The guide ensures that the journey progresses at an appropriate pace in an appropriate way and ultimately achieves a satisfactory outcome.

The qualifying programme is the start of what may become a lifelong journey that comprises more learning experiences, some good and some not so good, but all of which can be added to a personal store of knowledge. The main difference with the professional journey after qualification is that there is no guide. Each 'traveller', as a learning professional, has to be self-directed, planning and arranging different experiences for him or herself according to personal needs and interests. Some parts of the journey may suit immediate needs, others may be planned over a longer term as preparation for new roles or situations. This may entail academic study leading to a postgraduate award, or may take the form of other professional activity or experience. Some aspects of the career journey may not be planned at all. Opportunities will arise that will take you off a chosen course but offer you the means to try something new, and you will enjoy it for the moment. Sometimes you will recognise that learning is taking place, sometimes not. It is worth remembering that learning from *ad hoc* opportunities and experiences can be very meaningful and can even be enhanced using appropriate learning strategies. Whatever your career journey, there will be a need for ongoing learning to support it. Continuing professional development is necessary whether for maintaining competence in your current post or for developing your competence in preparation for a future post or role. Lifelong learning is therefore a feature of your professional working life.

Lifelong learning

Lifelong learning, according to Longworth & Davies, is 'the development of human potential through a continuously supportive process that stimulates and empowers individuals to acquire all the knowledge, values, skills and understanding they will require throughout their lifetimes and to apply them with confidence, creativity and enjoyment in all roles, circumstances and environments' (1996, p. 22). More simply, Knapper (1988, p. 105) described it as 'the ability to learn from life and throughout life' taking responsibility for one's own learning over the course of time. This involves learning to learn and developing an ability to learn autonomously and independently. In essence, the learner needs to take full responsibility for learning, including identifying and using those opportunities through which learning can occur. The process of *learning* in this sense is a personal responsibility and distinct from the process of *training* which depends on input from other people (Downs, 1993). Howells (1998) provided a helpful observation that lifelong learning is not about learning all the time but about treating learning as an everyday activity, returning to it throughout life to update and acquire new knowledge and skills.

Successful lifelong learning motivates individuals to participate further in learning but it has to be enjoyable if it is to be successful and of tangible benefit (Longworth & Davies, 1996). Benefit, of course, may be as much about a sense of personal fulfilment as about the prospect of increased income or better employment. The potential gains from learning may serve as motivators in the learning process even though the factors that motivate an individual may change over time. Longworth & Davies (1996) went so far as to suggest that there is more to lifelong learning than learning itself. There is a dimension to learning that can help to liberate the mind, to broaden personal horizons and to enable individuals to develop their unique potential to the full. This would suggest that, as with most things in life, the more effort you put in to something, the more you are likely to get out of it. So lifelong learning is likely to demand personal effort in order to reap any of the personal rewards.

Personal development

Personal development has been described as a process that enables individuals to generate their own strategies for the future (Callender, 1990). Personal development can be applied to any aspects of our lives, for example our health and fitness, our families and social encounters, and not just to the professional areas in which we work. The key, as Callender pointed out, is that whatever activities are pursued, they can expect to help the individual to develop new strengths and to overcome past weaknesses. Personal development may be linked to the development of the individual but can have a direct bearing on professional and organisational effectiveness, so it is important for employers to recognise and capitalise on those links. Personal and professional development can take place through a combination of planned events, the careful use of selected learning strategies, career moves and through unsolicited learning opportunities, representing both prospective and retrospective learning.

Professional learning

The first steps on the post-qualification career path may include a period of consolidation of learning and of applying new found knowledge under the supervision of, or in consultation with, a more experienced practitioner. Such experiences can provide opportunities for you to continue to learn in a less directed way and to further develop the confidence and competence you need for independent practice. For some of you, as newly qualified practitioners, your period of consolidation immediately after qualification may take place as part of a rotational scheme that enables you to gain experience in different specialty areas. Alternatively, some of you may opt for a post where you can develop more in-depth knowledge in a particular clinical area.

As your career starts to take shape, you may start to specialise and assume a wider level of responsibility for more complex or specialist cases, and may perhaps supervise other people. You may take on new roles and responsibilities in addition to that of practitioner and you may also have an opportunity to practise at a more advanced level with different service users. It is possible that, in the early days after qualification, much of your professional development will happen by chance rather than as a result of some pre-defined plan and may not be recorded in any formal way. Exceptions may be where you have access to a structured professional development programme of induction and development in professional practice. These schemes of one to two years' duration are normally organised by senior staff for newly qualified practitioners joining a service. Sometimes practitioners who are at an early stage of their career learn in a peer group, coming together for workshops, study days and lectures, and they may take part in other activities that enable them both to consolidate learning and to prepare for promotion. Many such schemes were originally designed to attract newly qualified practitioners to a service and were used as a strategy for retaining staff. While some schemes have been curtailed because of the loss of district coordinators or on account of service reorganisation, other schemes have been developed. Some are now multi-professional and some are accredited with a university and linked to an academic award. Where these schemes do exist they are generally very well received and well supported. They serve as a semi-structured learning system that encourages practitioners to take responsibility for their own learning and professional development.

Career stages and roles

The student

Your role development starts as you enter your professional education programme as a student in the role of learner-practitioner. The role of student is one that every qualified practitioner has experienced. As you progress through the educational programme you are exposed to a wide range of experiences and learning opportunities that help you to become socialised into your chosen profession. You learn about the profession's culture, language, and ways of working, and you become practised in making profession-specific contributions to health and social care and in making professional judgements when working with service users. The student role provides opportunities for personal development and professional growth, sometimes through routes that may be more difficult to access as a qualified practitioner just because of the pressure of work. Most of the learning experiences of students are structured within the framework of an agreed professional curriculum.

The student role provides opportunities to experiment, to put personal ideas into practice, to take risks within the relatively safe confines of supervised practice, to learn the consequences of actions, to learn from others, and to discriminate between good and less good practice. The student role is expected to function as a self-directed learner, learning through practice and reflection and through interaction with other people. The student is a learning role that has significant benefits over the practitioner role. However, in time, the student role ceases and you emerge as a practitioner. In this capacity you are expected to take on the role of employee within an organisation, working alongside other practitioners and with service users, and being responsible and accountable for all your professional activity.

The practitioner

The newly qualified practitioner can expect to spend the next 12–24 months consolidating learning in practice and developing confidence and competence. In a different way to the student, the practitioner is required to function as a self-directed and reflective practitioner who takes decisions based on independent professional judgement. This is not to say that all decisions must be taken independently of others. Part of the judgement will be to acknowledge personal limitations and to consult other people to obtain another professional opinion when this is felt to be necessary. This may be an opinion of an expert in the same field or of a practitioner in another field who has a different range of knowledge and skill. This in itself is a learning activity. Through interaction with peers, knowledge is developed that can be drawn upon in the future. Your role as a newly qualified practitioner involves learning about practice and about working in organisations. You will find out about areas of practice that you like and about those that you would like to learn more about,and at this point you may start to think about the direction of your career and your development needs.

Supervision and performance review

Your short and longer term development needs can partly be established formally through supervision and through a review of your performance at work. It is in your interest to have access to supervision and at least an annual performance review. For some professionals, your line manager may be a member of a different profession but that should not matter. What is important is for someone to set aside time on a regular basis to help work through issues with you. Time set aside for case supervision can often lead to discussions about gaps in knowledge and skills and short term professional development needs. Development needs may be specific to the profession or more general, such as development of management and leadership skills or skills for student supervision.

An individual performance review (IPR) or appraisal with a line manager can ensure that a more structured review of past performance and an evaluation of your current practice takes place and that your development plans for the future are identified and agreed. Your needs will be linked to the needs of the service and plans for the future. You are part of the organisation's workforce and therefore any plans for your professional development will need to fit into the wider plans for developing appropriate skills within the workforce. This ensures that service delivery meets organisational goals and user needs. It will help if you keep abreast of service developments so that you can match your career and educational needs with what is known to be required by the organisation. The arrangements for meeting your needs can be set out as a personal development plan (PDP) for you to take forward. Formally written, preferably as desired outcomes, these reviews and plans can form part of your professional portfolio.

Promotion and role extension

Once you are confident as a practitioner there are likely to be opportunities for you to move to different posts within the organisation and for you to gain additional clinical experience with different groups of service users. You might choose to take on other roles and responsibilities to complement your existing clinical role. For example, you might choose to develop skills as an educator, researcher or mentor, or you might become a committee member or a professional representative on a service-related project. New responsibilities can add a different dimension to the job. Role extension in this way is a horizontal move which does not involve promotion and is unlikely to attract additional financial reward but it can have other benefits in relation to personal and professional development. Developing competence in other clinical or service areas can broaden your interests and expertise, increase your self-esteem and personal confidence and help you prepare for career moves. It can offer opportunities for networking, increase your responsibilities, and in all can be personally satisfying and rewarding.

Eventually you may decide that you have sufficient confidence and competence to apply for promotion within your service or in another service. This usually means being prepared to accept a higher level of responsibility in areas of staff management, caseload management, or both. For those wishing to develop their career in this way, new responsibilities involving staff supervision and management and service administration allow practitioners to add to their repertoire of skills as they progress through their professional career. Career moves that lead to specialisation in an area of practice require the further development of specialist clinical skills. New roles in any respect are likely to require you to develop new knowledge and skills or to learn to apply your existing knowledge and skill in a different way. It is certainly advisable to seek some form of training or support to help you to undertake any new activity that carries with it a considerable increase in responsibility. Formal courses, often in-house, can assist you in this way. A mentor or coach can also help you to develop and apply new skills. Any development of this nature counts as learning and should be recorded as such.

Taking a job in another service can mean not only changing roles but also learning about new organisational structures and professional relationships. Moves may also result in a change in the balance of work undertaken in each role. For example, a practitioner who gains promotion may have to take additional responsibilities as a manager so the balance of practice versus managerial responsibilities shifts. Similarly, a senior practitioner who supervises more junior staff or extends the role to include research may have to adjust the time spent on the different aspects of the job. New responsibilities may require the practitioner to develop skills in a different domain or to develop existing skills to a different level of competence. Talking through the implications of change with a supervisor or mentor prior to career moves can be helpful. It can help you to decide what preparations you need and offer you support in adjusting to the changes. An action plan can be formulated in collaboration with your mentor which may indicate that some informal or a more formal educational programme may be beneficial to help you to develop new skills for the career move.

Lastly, but equally as important, you should remember that taking on additional responsibility will also change you. People will relate to you in a different way, particularly if the change has come about through promotion. This is something that is difficult to prepare for yet equally a part of your professional development. Having regular contact with a mentor and keeping a reflective diary are two strategies that might help you to manage this transition and capture the essence of your personal and professional development, particularly in the early stages of change. Increasingly, practitioners who are in more senior management positions are tending to seek regular personal consultations with management advisers or mentors who act as an external source of support and guidance. In these times of rapid change an adviser can provide the necessary support to help you keep stress levels under control. It should not be forgotten that all these are learning experiences. Even though they are a natural part of the job they still entail working through problems and issues that are new, and they are still an aspect of continuing professional development.

Strategies for role analysis and development

It should now be clear that you must take personal responsibility for determining the direction that your career should take. It is worth considering whether you want either to develop further expertise in a role that you already have and to work towards becoming a specialist or whether you just want to remain competent in your role by taking the steps necessary to keep up-to-date with changes in practice. You might also consider whether you want to change your role or to extend the role that you have. Perhaps you see your current position as one in which you will continue to practise for the foreseeable future or perhaps as a rung on a career ladder from where you hope to venture into new fields and develop different expertise as opportunities allow. The way that you plan to develop your skills will depend on how you see your current position and any future role and responsibilities.

Part of the strategy will entail looking critically at where you are now in your career, what career prospects you have and also taking stock of where your career fits into your private life and personal ambitions. You need to do this yourself even if you are working with a line manager and doing some of it through performance review. Your line manager may only take a narrow view of your professional development within the organisation and within the limits of service delivery, whereas you will take a broader view of where you are in your life and career. A mentor may help with either of these perspectives and provide a sounding board for other possibilities and opportunities within and beyond your profession. You first need to analyse the roles that you already have. List them and then ask:

- Am I happy with the roles I have or am I looking for something different?
- Where do these roles fit into the vision of my career?
- Do I need to rationalise and concentrate on the responsibilities of one or two key roles?
- Do I need to consolidate any of these roles or develop my skills?
- Do I need to extend the roles that I have in order to broaden my experience?
- Where am I going in my practice and in my career?
- What do I need to do to help me get there?

It is then necessary to consider all the options as well as the opportunities for role development, continuing professional development and personal career development. Opportunities may exist, for example, for a secondment, for taking on more responsibility, for taking an educational course, for carrying out project work, or for serving on a committee or working party. Any of these opportunities would provide for an expansion of roles. New roles can arise either through planned career moves or through unexpected opportunities that come your way. Opportunities may emerge through changes in personal or in organisational circumstances. If a new role is on offer it is worth considering the demands of the new role and the way in which it will impact on your existing roles and other aspects of your life. A role analysis may reveal your strengths, limitations and development needs, in other words, the factors that might affect your decision to move into the role and ultimately affect your success in it.

Taking stock of your professional development

Evaluating practice

As an integral part of professional practice you must take responsibility for reflecting on your own performance, for identifying your development needs and for taking steps to meet those needs. Needs may be as simple and short-term as the need to find out more about a particular medical condition. Alternatively, they may be more demanding and longer term, such as the need to develop skills in a particular technique, use of specialist equipment or in other aspects of practice, such as supervision or management.

Career development plans will emerge from a more detailed evaluation of your past experience, personal interests and future goals. Every so often you will need to take stock of your career to date and of whether your interests lie in taking on more responsibility and seeking promotion, or in developing and using your skills in a different area of practice, for example, in research, private consultancy, management or in education. Gaining promotion or moving from one area of work to another may entail purposely seeking opportunities to develop the appropriate skills and expertise in order for you to have every chance of success. Identification of strengths and limitations should indicate gaps in experience and skills that need to be developed for the new situation. A personal development plan to achieve personal goals would specify what you needed to do, how, and by when. It is important when setting out plans to think as creatively as possible. As already stated, professional development does not necessarily have to be costly and does not always entail attending courses. It is worth listing the knowledge, skills and expertise that you need to develop and then thinking of as many options as you can for addressing them. For example:

- Could someone locally teach you the necessary skills?
- Could you undertake some visits to develop your awareness of practice?
- Could you shadow someone?
- Could you arrange a secondment that will enable you to gain experience?

How much of the development plan can you take responsibility for yourself? For example, can you develop your knowledge base through a self-managed programme of study or do you really need external support and guidance? The hardest part is often setting out the learning goals and plans in such a way as to be achievable.

Professional development through secondments

One of the ways in which you can broaden your knowledge and expertise is to arrange a secondment in a different area of practice. A secondment normally entails being employed in another department, service or organisation for a set period of time, and with the agreement of your employer. Your current employer will normally continue to pay you but will be reimbursed by your new, temporary, employer. This gives you both continuity of employment and an opportunity to experience different kinds of work. The purpose of the secondment may either be to help the new employer in a task for which you have particular expertise, or to enable you to gain broader experience to develop you in your current role or to help you to prepare for a new role within the organisation. Often these arrangements are mutually beneficial. At the end of the agreed period of secondment you would normally return to your former place of work. A jobswap can also be considered as a way of developing two people in different roles with minimal disruption to service provision.

Agency work

A practitioner often takes up agency work because it serves their personal needs at the time. Some individuals thrive on agency work, others do it as a stop-gap for a short period between jobs or to test out whether they have the aptitude for a particular kind of work without committing to it. Agency work can be a flexible form of employment. You work when you choose to work, but it can also be unpredictable and without guarantee of suitable work at any point in time. It does, however, provide experience of work in different organisations and may ultimately lead to permanent employment in an organisation in which you have been working. Agency work is usually discouraged for newly qualified practitioners. It requires experience and the ability to work unsupervised, often without any form of introduction to the organisation. Agency work is a job without career prospects and without the normal conditions of employment such as annual leave, study leave, sick leave or maternity leave, so there is an element of risk. Anyone doing agency work is unlikely to have a personal development programme supported by the employing organisation. Career development moves and personal development plans will need to be constructed and directed by the agency workers themselves.

Taking a career break and returning to work

If you are considering taking a break in your professional career you may need to plan carefully how you can maintain your competence to practise, especially if you wish to return to practice at some later stage. Changes in legislation affecting the regulation of health professionals mean that evidence of competence may have to be provided before you can resume employment as a state registered practitioner. You may either need to plan a programme of continuing professional development while you are out of contact with health or social services or be prepared to undertake a return to practice course prior to re-entry into the profession. Keeping in contact with other practitioners in the field will help you keep abreast of some of the changes that are bound to occur.

Extended absence from service delivery may mean that your knowledge of the context of service provision and some of your professional knowledge and skills may become out-of-date or even obsolete. There will be a need for you to re-establish competence to practise in the current climate of health and social care and with current technology. You may need to take steps to regain competence by attending a structured return-to-practice scheme run by a university, local service or your professional body. Making a decision to return to practice can be extremely difficult. Very often it is confidence rather than ability that makes taking the first step so challenging. Some services offer return-to-practice schemes that allow for shadowing an experienced practitioner and include mentoring and supervision during the initial stages. This can help you to regain confidence in the workplace with the necessary support in the early stages.

Even though you may not be in contact with service users during your break, reading the profession's journal, or occasional attendance at professional development meetings or conferences may provide the basis for continuing professional development. A summary of activities and the learning resulting from them should form part of a portfolio for you to draw on as you return to practice. Once confidence is restored it should not be too difficult to demonstrate regained competence to practise.

Changing direction

Changing direction may mean moving to work in a different clinical field of practice, moving jobs, moving on to develop a new service or changing from working mainly with service users into an area of management, education, research or private practice. Any of these changes will require preparation. Plans and goals made explicit in a portfolio can help you to prepare for the changes by providing the structure for analysing your future development needs and detailing the action plan to be followed in order to meet them. A portfolio of evidence that you have the appropriate experience and have prepared yourself for the new role may support your application for the career move.

The changing nature of employment

The employment market has changed considerably as Handy (1996) has consistently pointed out. Handy does not necessarily see this change as disadvantageous but more as opening up opportunities for taking alternative career paths. Where employees might previously have expected to serve in an organisation for a number of years and progress to positions of increasing responsibility, there is now a trend for short-term contracts and more uncertainty in employment. There are flatter organisational structures with fewer opportunities for career progression. To counteract this trend, Handy sees the advent of a 'portfolio' culture where an individual accumulates evidence of skills and abilities and sells services to those who wish to buy. While this mode of operating gives the individual less certainty about employment it does offer more control over what he or she accepts as work. The portfolio career does, however, necessitate continuous updating of professional skills and requires the practitioner to maintain an awareness and responsiveness to changes in all aspects of the environment.

Lifelong learning is a concept that has to be associated with the new career pattern. This point is also argued by Barnett (1994, p. 182) who urges us to think beyond achieving and maintaining competence. Society *is* changing, and individuals must go on learning and renewing their knowledge. They need to develop new skills to enhance productive capacity or address new concepts as the definition of their professional field changes. Almost certainly it will rely on self-evaluation of professional practice and learning to adapt to changing circumstances. Outdated practices will have to be discarded and new areas of responsibility accepted as a necessary part of professional life. This includes learning to cope with changes in your life circumstances (McGivney, 1993). It is worth remembering here that the Institute of Health Services Management defines continuous professional development as 'the individual ... taking responsibility for the development of his/her own career by systematically analysing development needs, identifying and using appropriate methods to meet these needs and regularly reviewing achievements compared against personal and career objectives' (Coates, 1997). It is recognised here that each individual must take control of and manage his or her career. Employment trends are not so stable that this can be ignored.

References

Ashton, J. (1992) Continuing education: study of the professional development of therapists. Unpublished PhD thesis, University of Exeter.

Barnett, R. (1994) *The Limits of Competence*. Society for Research into Higher Education and Open University Press, Buckingham.

Callender, P. (1990) Why personal development workshops? In *Self-development in Organisations* (M. Pedlar, J. Burgoyne, T. Boydell & G. Welshman, eds). McGraw-Hill, London.

Clyne, S. (1995) *Continuing Professional Development Perspectives on CPD in Practice*. Kogan Page, London.

Coates, M. (1997) Much more than this... *Health Management* **Sept**, 10–13.

Downs, S. (1993) Developing learning skills in vocational learning. In *Culture and Processes of Adult Learning* (M. Thorpe, R. Edwards & A. Hanson, eds). Routledge, London.

Eraut, M. (1994) *Developing Professional Knowledge and Competence*. The Falmer Press, London.

Haines, P. (1997) Professionalization through CPD: is it realistic for achieving our goals? *British Journal of Therapy and Rehabilitation* **4**, 428–47.

Handy, C. (1996) *Beyond Certainty*. Arrow Business Books, London.

Hollis, V. (1997) Practice portrayed: an exploration of occupational therapy clinical skills and their development. Unpublished PhD thesis, University of Exeter.

Howells, K. (1998) Learning is for life. *The Lecturer* **July**, 13.

Knapper, C. (1988) Technology and lifelong learning. In *Developing Student Autonomy in Learning* (D. Boud, ed). 2nd edn. Kogan Page, London.

Longworth, N. & Davies, W.K. (1996) *Lifelong Learning*. Kogan Page, London.

McGivney, V. (1993) Participation and non-participation a review of the literature. In *Adult Learners, Education and Training* (R. Edwards, S. Sieminski & D. Zeldin, eds). Routledge, London.

Chapter 5

Competence: Maintenance and Development

What constitutes competence?

The premise on which this book is written is that there is a need for practitioners to take steps to maintain their competence through continuing professional development, not only for their own competence in practice but also for ongoing state registration. Codes of Ethics and Professional Conduct outline expectations of practitioners that they will offer up to date health care to service users and practise safely and effectively at all times. New statutory requirements implemented under the Health Act 1999 are set to strengthen these expectations by placing obligations on members of the professions allied to medicine to take steps to remain competent to practise. The new legislation reinforces the Government's agenda for improving quality in health care through competent and effective practice (Department of Health, 1998).

In the past state registration has assumed, possibly unreliably, a state of competence that remained steady over time but the notion of enduring competence is now no longer being taken for granted, indeed it is being challenged. Evidence of continued competence may now be needed for re-registration. Maintaining a basic level of competence that satisfies the conditions of state registration is the first requirement. This is essential for practice as it ensures that the public will be protected. Developing competence to a higher level of expertise is likely to give added value to service delivery by enhancing a practitioner's capacity to practise in his or her profession within a constantly changing health care environment. Competence development also helps to prepare practitioners for employment in specialist areas of practice, for single-handed practice and for supervising and coaching others in more junior or student roles.

In order for judgements to be made about the state of competence, however, some interpretation of the term is necessary. Competence is a notoriously difficult concept to define and can be open to many interpretations. A definition is essential, however, if distinctions are to be made between 'competence', 'incompetence', 'lack of competence' and 'not yet competent'. The implications of incompetence and lack of competence could be very serious for an individual whose level of competence is called into question under new statutory arrangements. Explicit criteria against which competence is to be judged would therefore seem to be crucial.

Some definitions

General and more concrete definitions of competence indicate that it refers to the ability of an individual to perform a particular activity to a prescribed standard – the ability to perform in the workplace to the standards required in employment. Competence, defined in this way, therefore has both a personal and situational dimension, as Hollis (1997) has acknowledged. Barnett (1994, p. 71) claimed that 'to say of an individual that he is competent is to assert that his actions are coming up to a standard'. Many academics, however, including Barnett himself, have recognised that such a definition of competence is simplistic and inadequate. Eraut (1994, p. 166), for example, added some positive and negative dimensions, offering definitions of competence respectively as capable of 'getting the job done' and 'adequate but less than excellent'. The implication with the latter definition is that someone who is more than adequate, or even excellent, would still be considered competent, suggesting that different levels of competence can be described. The novice to expert continuum (Dreyfus & Dreyfus, 1986) validates this notion of levels of competence, but whilst it may be possible to distinguish between these different levels, determining the line between competent and incompetent, or determining what constitutes lack of competence, could still be difficult.

Fish & Twinn (1997) drawing on the work of Carr (1993) argued in more abstract terms that competence is about the capacity to exercise principled judgement, the capacity to adapt and improvise rather than merely the ability to follow rules and routines. However credible this argument, the definition may be insufficiently detailed for the purpose of making judgements about lack of competence or incompetence for continued state registration. The irony is that things that go wrong in practice tend often to stem from inappropriate, a misuse of, or a lack of, professional judgement where the principles underpinning decisions taken cannot be articulated. Decisions taken can be challenged in relation to the principles commonly used by a competent practitioner.

Another question to be considered is this. Should the definition of competence or level of clinical expertise be the same for the purpose of maintaining state registration for a qualified practitioner as for a qualifying student who has just become eligible to apply for state registration? Statutory requirements expect a basic level of competence of everyone on the state register. Protection of the public is assured on the premise that all qualified practitioners can operate at least to the basic level of competence defined for a newly qualifying practitioner. Matuscak (1983) provided a helpful definition of competence that might be considered more relevant to health professionals. Matuscak suggested that competence is:

'the ability of the about-to-graduate student to integrate knowledge, judgement, affective behaviour and professional skills in such a way that they meet or exceed the standards of professional functioning that are demanded by a professional body deemed qualified to set those standards'.

This definition acknowledges judgement and the fact that competence for everyone has to be assessed at the point of entry to a profession but it also implies that competence is in a time warp, a constant steady state, where the notion of what constitutes competence need not change. Hollis (1997) on the other hand pointed out that competence is unlikely to be static and suggested that it is context-specific. She advocated Day's (1995) definition of competence which is given as the possession ...

'of the necessary skills, knowledge, attitudes, understanding and experience required to perform in professional and occupational roles to a satisfactory standard within the workplace'.

This would suggest that as the nature of the workplace changes so will practice, and thus what constitutes competence to practise in that environment. This reflects what actually happens in practice because health care policies, systems and structures all have an impact on a practitioner's work. Any changes to them result in organisational changes that can have a domino effect on the nature of service provision and on practitioners' work. The latter definition, however, addresses performance rather than judgement – outcome rather than process – so may still have some limitations as a definition for assessing the continued competence of health care practitioners. It should be noted, however, that the Government has advocated partnership arrangements with the professional and regulatory bodies to monitor and support CPD initiatives within the context of clinical governance (Department of Health, 1999). The expectation is that, regardless of the detail of definition, there will be a commonly agreed agenda for maintaining competent professionals in the workplace through collaboration.

Functions of the professional bodies

Professional bodies already take steps to support the membership in the process of maintaining professional standards, working collaboratively with the statutory regulatory body to protect the public. This entails ensuring that professional qualifying programmes meet required standards and that the practitioners qualifying from those programmes are competent to practise in their profession. The development and assessment of competence is an explicit aspect of approved educational programmes leading to eligibility for state registration, although the lack of consensus about competence (see above) might suggest that this could be a very subjective process. Professional bodies also encourage the membership to develop professionally in order to enhance their practice and thus the service delivered to the public. In addition, professional bodies advise members about the implications of change in environment, policy and other aspects of professional practice. They may propose an agenda for working harmoniously with changes whilst preserving the quality and value of the professional contribution to practice.

Professional bodies also aim to protect the membership from exploitation and offer guidance on good practice. For example, it is generally advocated that newly qualified professionals still have to consolidate their learning and would normally expect to do so in practice under the supervision of, or in consultation with, an experienced practitioner. Therefore newly qualified practitioners are not normally deployed to deal with the most complex cases or to use complex techniques or equipment. Practice under supervision is normally recommended before the practitioner takes responsibility for more challenging work. In some professions, additional qualifications or endorsements to qualifications may be required. More demanding or complex jobs requiring a higher level of skill and competence therefore normally remain in the domain of the more experienced practitioner.

Fitness for purpose and fitness for practice

The notions of *fitness for purpose* and *fitness for practice* are commonly used for describing, respectively, the capability of the employee in the workplace and the capacity of the individual to practise in his or her profession. These are useful distinctions but still embrace different levels of capability and capacity. Fitness for purpose, for example, could be applied both to qualities expected for employment in posts requiring basic levels of expertise and for positions requiring specialist knowledge and skills in the same profession. Likewise, fitness for practice could rest somewhere on a continuum from competent to expert practitioner. Competence, and continuing competence, are likely to be judged in relation to both fitness for purpose and fitness for practice at a basic level. Additionally, problems still remain because what is judged to be an acceptable level of competence or 'fitness' will change over time. The report *Improving the Effectiveness of Quality Assurance in Non-medical Health Care Education and Training* (an initiative jointly sponsored by the NHS Executive, Higher Education Quality Council and Yorkshire Regional Health Authority in 1996) pointed out that judgements about fitness for practice derive from professional notions about the scope and nature of practice which tend to change through time in an evolutionary or incremental way. This reinforces the idea of competence and context being interrelated.

Context and competence – further considerations

Judgements about who is qualified to undertake specialist work are normally made by employers. They would be expected to take professional advice from an acknowledged 'expert' member of the profession about the relative competence of an applicant for more specialised clinical work. It would be up to employers to deploy practitioners appropriately and to demand (and verify) that an employee has the additional specific, higher level skills deemed necessary for the post. Maintenance of competence at this level would then be necessary for continued employment, for ongoing service provision and for protection of the public.

The maintenance of competence at this higher, specialist level would thus be essential for retaining a senior position in employment and for carrying out the complex duties associated with the job. The distinction to be made here is that maintenance of competence at this higher level is necessary for employment entailing complex work, but may not be necessary for maintaining state registration. Benchmark standards, however, may be used to validate higher levels of competence or competence in areas that support practice, such as management. The professional body and the statutory regulatory body can validate competence to practise at the entry gate to a profession but currently the employer is expected to ensure that each employee has the competence to fulfil the job for which he or she is employed, whatever the level and complexity of the work.

Taking account of various definitions, competence may be thought of as being both general and context-specific. Competence that is specific to one situation may not necessarily be transferable to another. In other words, a practitioner may be considered to be competent in relation to a particular environment but not to others, although this would contradict the argument that competence implies the capacity to make judgements in the context of changing circumstances. The argument would be that, if the environment changes, the change may affect the performance of the practitioner and the outcome for the service user. The environment includes political, economic, sociological and technological factors that affect service delivery. Practitioners, in collaboration with their employers, have a responsibility to maintain an awareness of the environment in which they practise to ensure their continuing competence in that environment and in the light of changing circumstances. Principled practice must therefore involve constantly testing principles in new situations and ensuring that reflections on practice provide a continuous flow of information that will support future practice and guide any changes required.

As an example, we can reflect on the changes that occurred as a result of the implementation of the National Health Service and Community Care Act 1990. The move to community care changed the context and nature of health care delivery and brought about enormous changes in the practice of many of the professions allied to medicine. Practitioners had to develop new ways of working and confidence in different roles in the community, without the immediate support of facilities in a large institution. Being proactive in the light of change and taking the initiative to learn how to operate in a new environment enabled practitioners to continue to function in new areas of service provision and to maintain an effective service. During this process, competence shifted in relation to the environment, because skills had to be used in different ways or new skills developed, but there was also an expectation that health professionals would take this in their stride and accommodate the changes. In future, other changes can be expected as Primary Care Trusts (PCTs) are established under the statutory framework of the Health Act 1999 and as clinical governance and evidence-based practice take a foothold. It is possible that some practices will be eliminated, others expanded and new ways of working adopted. Competence in context may need to be redefined.

Developing competence

Competence cannot merely be associated with skill development as Barnett (1994) and Fish & Twinn (1997) have argued. Competence in professional practice has to include the judgements needed to use skills in new and different situations. Fish & Twinn (1997, p. 48) pointed out the difference between the terms 'competence' and 'competency'. They defined competence as the capacity to make professional judgements according to the situation, and competency as the operation of predetermined skills developed through training. Barnett (1994, p. 73) made it quite clear that today's competency is not tomorrow's, so that anyone who is currently deemed competent must be able to adapt effectively to the changes in the environment that affect practice in order to maintain the state of competence over time. Competent performance is therefore more than the operation of technical skills. It embraces both knowledge *and* abilities (Eraut, 1994). It involves professional judgements that draw on a specialised knowledge base integrated with knowledge from a store of experiences from which learning has already occurred. Continuing professional development must therefore acknowledge the complexity and dynamics of practice and involve more than just a theoretical knowledge base.

We can conclude that the notion of competence has to embrace the capacity of practitioners to modify what they do within a changing world (Barnett, 1994). Competence is therefore not a static feature but a dynamic one where there is a close relationship between competence and context. The nature of competence changes as the environment changes and this has a bearing on the activities that help to sustain competence, such as continuing professional development. Remaining static and resisting or ignoring change may affect the ability of practitioners to function adequately in new situations. It has been estimated that knowledge and skills can become out of date at the rate of about half of a professional's knowledge every five years (Ashton, 1992), so competence diminishes. Keeping up to date with change, and foreseeing the consequences of change, enable practitioners to take steps to prepare themselves for working in new contexts and for maintaining the competence to do so.

Lastly, for those who have taken on new roles and responsibilities associated with their profession in areas of management, research or education, difficulties can arise in the interpretation of competence for the purposes of continuing professional development for state registration. As Eraut (1994, p. 167) argued, 'individuals change the scope of their competence throughout their professional career, moving into more specialist work, into new or developing areas of practice or taking on managerial or educational responsibilities, so the parameters of competence change'. Dimensions of competence for state registration must therefore be sensitive enough to respect and reflect these changes because they are a natural progression and allow professionals to enhance their roles and develop their careers. We should not lose sight of the fact that all these different roles have a part to play within the NHS.

In a report for physiotherapists Powell (1997) proposed a model of CPD that differentiated between newly qualified practitioners, those returning to practise, and experienced and specialist practitioners but he acknowledged that the model would be dependent on the new legislation being flexible enough to accommodate different membership categories. The proposed model was underpinned by the potential of benchmark standards established for the workplace that would provide reference points against which judgements about quality might be made. Powell (1999) later suggested that standards for each profession could be determined and developed by the relevant professional body and the statutory regulatory body to reflect 'competence' or 'fitness' for professional practice before and after qualification. Those institutions providing programmes leading to professional qualification would assess students' fitness for practice, using the relevant benchmark standards for the point of qualification. After qualification, other standards would be used that reflect the enhanced capacity of individuals to work, for example, in areas of management. As yet it is not clear whether this model will be supported. Whatever the model eventually adopted, individuals are likely to be required to demonstrate continuing competence for re-registration with the regulatory body.

Competence –whose responsibility?

Until recently, the locus of responsibility for the maintenance of competence has not been clear. According to Eraut (1994, p. 159) 'the public expects a qualified professional to be competent in the discharge of normal professional tasks and duties'. This would imply that the individual is primarily responsible for the maintenance of his or her professional skills and knowledge so as to be able to carry out duties competently. This tends to be reinforced in Codes of Professional Conduct. On the other hand, organisations delivering health and social care have increasingly had to take responsibility for providing services as efficiently and effectively as possible. Managers are expected to employ competent staff to undertake the organisation's duties and to ensure that employees continue to practise 'to the current accepted approved practice of reasonable practitioners in that field' (Dimond, 1997, p. 327). Ensuring the ongoing competence of the workforce must be in the employers' interests in order to minimise the risk of harm to the public and unnecessary claims for compensation. Employer support for programmes that maintain the competence of the workforce is therefore crucial. It could also be argued that ensuring that the workforce remains competent and able to provide services efficiently and effectively is a critical factor for retaining a stable and motivated workforce. Employers would thus need to be proactive in maintaining a competent workforce through staff development in order to achieve effective service delivery and not just as a token for avoiding failure.

To ensure the continued safety of employees and the public they serve employers are statutorily obliged to provide training for their employees (Health and Safety Executive, 1992), but unless mandated to do so, employers may not take equal responsibility for ensuring the ongoing competence of the workforce even though it might seem necessary for staff retention and quality assurance purposes. Ovretveit (1992) argued that employees must be knowledgeable and skilled in the range of techniques necessary to assess and treat service users and that they should be able to use the techniques properly. Adequate education and training is therefore essential. Education and training is also necessary for staff who are expected to take on new duties so that work can be carried out safely and effectively. After all, it tends to be the employer who manipulates the work environment and context of practice, bringing about changes that it expects employees to follow through. There seems to be a value attributed to different kinds of education and training. As Eraut (1994) noted, organisations might support continuing professional development for the purpose of organisational change but might not support it for improving the quality of professional practice, thus taking a rather short-sighted and fragmented approach to maintaining and improving service quality.

The quality of professional practice may be left to the profession alone to determine, monitored to some extent through organisational audit. This does mean that any initiative for continuing professional development to improve professional practice or the quality of service delivery may be taken independently by employees rather than collaboratively within a cohesive strategy for service improvement. Audits may bring to light difficulties or deficits in service provision and may help to justify staff development programmes, but this is a piece-meal, reactive approach to CPD rather than a coordinated and proactive one. Continuing professional development can of course help to motivate and retain staff but, as Brennan (1992) observed, if employers are to make a financial commitment to staff development they expect to see some return for the investment in terms of benefits for service users. Any staff development, collective or individual, must therefore be linked to goals for improvements in service provision.

More recently, the Government has made it clear that CPD is a shared responsibility between the individual and employer, with regulatory and professional bodies playing their part to help set and maintain standards. In future, CPD activity can expect to support the clinical governance agenda and underpin service developments. Clinical guidelines produced by the National Institute for Clinical Effectiveness (NICE) will serve as a focus for CPD and employers will be expected to align training funds to local service objectives (Department of Health, 1999). Those health professionals who work in the NHS can expect to be part of a workforce that is able, willing and supported in its efforts to maintain competence and to develop practice.

Despite this, it is still important for individuals to monitor their own performance and take steps to maintain competence for state registration. Continuing professional development supports the professional career, not just the job, and not all health professionals work in the National Health Service to which many of these policies primarily apply. Maintaining competence for state registration is an ethical, professional and individual responsibility, and must be acknowledged as such. The responsibility of employers is to ensure that each member of staff is competent in the job and remains so, is deployed appropriately, and that CPD not only underpins current work, but also any future changes in roles, responsibilities and service development.

Competence and clinical governance

Recent Government literature has required us to rethink the need and responsibility for maintaining competence and for practising effectively. As mentioned earlier in this chapter, the National Health Service and Community Care Act 1990 had an impact on the way in which practitioners worked, requiring them to develop expertise that would allow them to deliver more services in the community. This trend is set to continue. TheWhite Paper *The New NHS: modern, dependable* (1997) proposed that greater focus be placed on services provided through primary care and the Health Act 1999 now places these proposals in a statutory framework. In the proposed changes, the notion of clinical governance was introduced. This will increasingly have an effect on the way in which practitioners work and how they monitor and audit their performance. Clinical governance is described in the White Paper (1997, p. 82) as 'actions to ensure that risks are avoided, adverse events are rapidly detected, openly investigated and lessons learned, good practice is rapidly disseminated and systems are in place to ensure continuous improvements in clinical care'. These are obviously measures to ensure effective service provision through competent performance and the evaluation of practice. All practitioners, teams and services are being required to take steps to ensure the ongoing improvement in professional practice and service provision. Collective competence is therefore also subject to assessment.

The directives expect responsibility to be taken at different levels:

- Individuals must take responsibility for the quality of their own clinical performance
- Professional self-regulation is required
  - to maintain and improve standards
  - to be responsive to changing service needs
  - to ensure public accountability
- Corporate governance is necessary for organisations to ensure
  - that quality is at the core of service delivery
  - that local arrangements are in place for monitoring performance and improving quality
  - accountability for their effective operation, not only financially but also in terms of quality.

Cook (1998) provided a useful summary of the five activities that form the basis of clinical governance:

(1) *Research and development*
   - primary research
   - implementation of research findings
   - critical appraisal of research evidence

(2) *Risk management*
   - health and safety maintenance
   - clinical risk assessment
   - staff training
   - policy/procedure development

(3) *Quality initiatives*
   - continuing professional development
   - standard setting
   - complaints handling
   - user involvement

(4) *Clinical effectiveness initiatives*
   - standard setting
   - evidence reviews
   - production of clinical guidelines

(5) *Audit*
   - criterion-based audit
   - significant event audit

It is clear from this analysis that these activities should promote service effectiveness through service-related development activity but the analysis also helps to identify where gaps in knowledge and skills might occur that need to be addressed by individuals or teams.

Filling the gaps and undertaking development activities can be construed as learning that can form the basis of continuing professional development. This means that initiatives for clinical governance should also result in learning and continuing professional development. Learning that results from development activity needs to be identified so that new knowledge informs future practice. Learning is related both to context and to the quality of service provision. Documented in an appropriate form, this learning can provide evidence of professional development. Thus a link can be seen between clinical governance and continuing professional develpment, as well as between context and competence to practise.

References

Ashton, J. (1992) Continuing education: study of the professional development of therapists. Unpublished PhD thesis, University of Exeter.

Barnett, R. (1994) *The Limits of Competence*. Society for Research into Higher Education and Open University Press, Buckingham.

Brennan, A. (1992) Analysing mandatory continuing education. *Nursing Standard* **6**, 29–41.

Carr, D (1993) Questions of competence. Cited in D. Fish & S. Twinn (1997) *Quality Clinical Supervision in the Health Care Professions*. Butterworth Heinemann, Oxford.

Cook, R. (1998) Picture in profile. *Health Service Journal* **108**, 26–7.

Day, M. (1995) Putting vocational training into practice. Cited in V. Hollis (1997) Practice portrayed: an exploration of occupational therapy clinical skills and their development. Unpublished PhD thesis, University of Exeter.

Department of Health (1998) *A First Class Service – Quality in the New NHS*. Department of Health, Leeds.

Department of Health (1999) *Continuing Professional Development: Quality in the New NHS*. Department of Health, Leeds.

Dimond, B.C. (1997) *Legal Aspects of Occupational Therapy*. Blackwell Science, Oxford.

Dreyfus, H.L. & Dreyfus, S.E. (1986) *Mind over Machine: The Power of Human Intuition and Expertise in the Era of the Computer*. Blackwell, Oxford.

Eraut, M. (1994) *Developing Professional Knowledge and Competence*. The Falmer Press, London.

Fish, D. & Twinn, S. (1997) *Quality Clinical Supervision in the Health Care Professions: Principled Approaches to Practice*. Butterworth Heinemann, Oxford.

Health and Safety Executive (1992) *Manual Handling – Guidance on Regulations*. HMSO, London.

Hollis, V. (1997) Practice portrayed: an exploration of occupational therapy clinical skills and their development. Unpublished PhD thesis, University of Exeter.

Matuscak, R. (1983) Criteria, purposes and methods for evaluating the clinical competence of students in the allied health professions. Cited in M. Ernest and H. Polatajko (1996) Performance evaluation of occupational therapy students: a validity study. *Canadian Journal of Occupational Therapy* **53**, 265–71.

Ovretveit, J. (1992) *Health Service Quality: An Introduction to Quality Methods for Health Services*. Blackwell Science, Oxford.

Powell, A. (1997) *A Framework for Continuing Professional Development*. Chartered Society of Physiotherapy, London.

Powell, A. (1999) Assuring the Quality of Health Care Education and Training. Unpublished Interim Report to the Department of Health, Leeds.

Chapter 6
Equipped to Learn

Learning to learn as a dimension of competence

Career development requires individuals to build on their knowledge and skills to develop their level of competence from that gained during their initial professional education. As has been discussed, competence embraces many professional and technical skills and personal qualities necessary for effective practice. It also has to include skills for effective learning so that professional development can continue to take place. Personal, professional and technical skills are essential to practice but being able to learn is essential for maintaining practice skills, for continuing professional development and for taking on new roles. Competence to learn should therefore be integral to competence to practise.

Professional programmes leading to qualification are part of a continuum of education seen within the context of lifelong learning. It is important to remember that lifelong learning actually starts pre-school, and continues through the formal years of education, both inside and outside schools and colleges, into adulthood. This learning provides the foundation skills required to operate and survive within society. After compulsory education the adult has a choice to continue to learn in an educational institution or to develop skills through work and other life experiences, or to do both. The mode and pace of learning and the structure in which learning takes place are likely to differ for each individual, nevertheless learning will be ongoing. It is up to the individual how learning experiences are captured and used, and the extent to which learning progresses. This is likely to depend on an individual's capacity and motivation to learn, level of commitment to self-development, and the degree to which skills and strategies for learning are in place.

In a professional forum it is easy to think of professional education as being the way forward. Yet personal development is an important form of learning that has much to contribute to professional development. Personal development comes from a range of experiences through the roles we play in life, holidays that we take, books that we read, people that we meet and talk to, and many other planned and unexpected personal experiences. We participate in lifelong learning as we participate in everyday life even though we may not even recognise that learning is taking place. Knowledge and personally constructed meaning from encounters are stored for later use. Personal learning includes developing confidence, self-esteem and the skills of communication that assist with the building of rapport and working relationships with other people.

The responsibility for lifelong learning as a professional is rather different. It has to be a conscious commitment and undertaken seriously and systematically. It is a professional responsibility that helps to ensure that the most up-to-date service can be provided to the public based on sound principles and evidence of good practice. This meets professional ethical requirements and expectations of other people with regard to safe, competent and effective practice. However, for learning to be effective, skills for learning, and not just skills for practice, have to be acquired and refined. Many professional education programmes now use teaching, learning and assessment strategies that not only facilitate learning but that also provide students with strategies for their ongoing educational and professional development. In this way, the newly qualified practitioner leaves university having been socialised into his or her chosen profession, having developed adequate professional knowledge and skills for competent perfor- mance, having an understanding of professional principles, having developed reasoning skills for making competent professional judgements, and having developed the skills for ongoing development.

Competence in learning is about having a positive attitude to education, about taking the initiative to learn, about being open to new methods of practice, and about seizing learning opportunities and working with new ideas and concepts to improve professional performance. It is about developing the skills to question and reflect on practice, to evaluate one's own performance and to accept and respond to constructive feedback. It is about practising and refining skills, knowing when and where to seek help and guidance and knowing how to use learning resources effectively. Skills related to learning that are developed initially as a student are likely to include the ability to:

- Search for, select, analyse and interpret information to support learning
- Use guided observation
- Use skills of reflection and critical appraisal
- Set and work towards meeting learning goals and objectives
- Discriminate between different information and make judgements
- Learn through problem-oriented, problem-based or solution-focused methods
- Use a learning contract
- Practise reflectively, possibly using reflective diaries or logs
- Learn experientially
- Engage in and manage project work
- Investigate practice and carry out research
- Learn independently and through self-managed study
- Apply new learning to practice situations

The ability to locate and use different resources effectively, including libraries, written material and experts in the field, is part of the programme of skill development. It can easily be forgotten that these skills have already been developed during initial professional education and can be drawn upon for the process of continuing professional development. As Gratton & Pearson (1994, p. 86) have pointed out, if we provide individuals with a greater capacity to learn from the widest variety of opportunities we are empowering them to be in greater command of their destiny. The skills for learning are the foundation skills that help individuals to develop practice-related skills and to prepare for new roles.

Learning to develop competence

In pre-registration professional education it is common for programmes to be structured to allow students to develop skills for independent practice over time. Teaching and learning strategies enable students to take progressively greater levels of responsibility for their learning, both in the academic environment and in clinical and fieldwork situations in order to prepare them for their role as an independent practitioner. Of course, the term 'independent' has to be seen in a comparative sense since students do not practise independently. Even newly qualified practitioners are initially likely to practise under the supervision of a more experienced therapist while consolidating their learning in practice. As competence and confidence grow, so practitioners are able to assume greater levels of responsibility for independent practice and for practice in more complex circumstances.

The acquisition of competence to practise could be described as the incremental development of competence through different stages and levels. Dreyfus & Dreyfus (1986) described five developmental stages on a continuum from novice to expert. Dowie and Elstein (1988, p. 95) presented the key features of these five stages which have been summarised in Table 6.1. The inexperienced practitioner relies more on analysis for reasoning whereas the expert uses intuitive processes. Intuitive performance will initially be poor, but can be improved with practice. Overall, however, intuition tends to result in better performance because it enables practitioners to deal with unexpected and novel situations to which the normal rules of practice (as used in analytical approaches) do not apply.

It is also worth reminding ourselves here that in Chapter 5 we referred to competence as being related to context. The way in which competence development is addressed by Table 6.1 seems to pay no attention to context. Although we can draw on theoretical models to start examining competence and to show that it develops incrementally through a learning process, there are innumerable facets of that process that indicate that competence development is not as simple as the table might imply.

In assessing competence, it may be found that selected areas of a therapist's practice are below that expected of a competent practitioner. In other areas, however, the therapist may be proficient or even expert. It is important to be aware of the fact that we may be competent to different degrees in different areas of our jobs. It is possible that on self-evaluation, a practitioner might consider

Table 6.1 Stages of professional development.

Stage of development	Characteristics of the individual
Expert	Has clear vision based on reflective experience Has an intuitive grasp of situations Makes decisions intuitively
Proficient	Has a sense of direction and vision Sees situations holistically, not as components Discriminates between important and less important information Perceives situations intuitively Makes strategic decisions analytically Modifies action as situation changes
Competent	Combines perception and action Thinks analytically about whole situation Plans deliberately and consciously Tends to follow some procedures routinely
Advanced beginner	Is learning to distinguish between sets of information Applies other people's rules to practice
Novice	Thinks analytically about components of practice Refers to guiding principles Follows other people's rules

him or herself to be an expert in some areas of practice but only competent in others. He or she may be an expert in clinical practice yet only proficient or competent as a manger or clinical supervisor. Competence assessment should help a practitioner to determine which areas of his or her job require further development.

Developing competence entails:

- Knowing how competence is defined and understood
- Being able to assess one's personal competence to practise in different areas
- Identifying gaps or limitations in knowledge and skills and in their application in practice
- Planning a programme of activity to develop a higher level of competence in selected areas of practice
- Knowing how to find and use the resources that will assist in personal development
- Monitoring and evaluating performance in respect of changing personal and situational circumstances

Fish & Twinn (1997) asserted that experience of practice is essential for the development of competence and that learning depends on effective skills of reflection, a concept discussed later in the book.

Developing reasoning skills

According to Higgs & Jones (1995) health care practitioners have several key responsibilities:

- To practise in a manner that demonstrates professional autonomy, competence and accountability
- To engage in lifelong learning
- To contribute to the development of the profession's knowledge base

All of these responsibilities subsume the ability to learn and to use new learning in an effective way for the benefit of service users, the profession and the individual practitioner. In order to manage these responsibilities, health professionals need to learn to reason effectively. Having the capacity to reason effectively not only promotes effective practice but it also enables the practitioner to manage complex and changing information in the practice environment, an argument supported by Fish & Twinn (1997) in their debate on competence.

Clinical reasoning, defined as 'the thinking and decision-making processes integral to clinical practice', has been said to be the foundation of professional practice (Higgs & Jones, 1995). It is concerned with the ability to address and resolve clinical or care management problems encountered in professional practice using carefully selected strategies that take account of all facets of the service user's story and personal situation. Clinical reasoning occurs within several contexts:

- The immediate personal context of the service user
- The clinical or functional problem experienced and the setting in which it is being addressed
- The personal and professional framework of the health care practitioner
- The broad context of health and social care
- The complex context of professional decision-making in practice

Clinical reasoning is therefore a complex activity that can only be refined with practice.

The development of initial clinical reasoning skills is seen as essential for those seeking a professional qualification and much literature has been produced to support teaching and learning about the process at undergraduate level. But as Dutton (1995) remarked, no one expects a student to develop all the required clinical reasoning skills at once. Understanding the full depth and potential of clinical reasoning and gaining expertise in it is an ongoing process of discovery that occurs throughout the professional career (Higgs, 1997). An initial understanding of clinical reasoning can be developed prior to qualification and skills can be rehearsed in clinical practice, but this is only the beginning. A conscious effort needs to be made after qualification to continue the learning process associated with the development of reasoning skills, and thus with the development of proficiency and expertise.

Higgs (1997) noted that the clinical setting provides the opportunity for students to develop their knowledge base by discovering meaning and by endeavouring to make sense of learning experiences in practice. In the process of learning to reason, students question what they are learning, reflect on their thoughts and actions, explore the validity and effects of different ways of achieving goals, experiment with new ideas, and discuss thoughts and experiences with others. Learning to do this establishes a pattern of activity that will continue during professional life. This is therefore one way in which qualified practitioners might be expected to develop and refine their reasoning skills after qualification. It is only by being exposed to and working with different clinical problems and scenarios that a mental store of experiences will develop as reference points for subsequent problem-solving during practice. Post-qualifying experience is therefore essential to the further development of clinical reasoning skills but this learning has to be nurtured. Initially skills are developed during the qualifying educational programme where there is a structure for learning, but after qualification practitioners are responsible for the continuation of their own learning. Skills for learning therefore need to be refined so that learning in practice and through practice can be maximised for the ongoing development of clinical skills.

Depth and breadth of skill development

The novice-to-expert continuum helps us to understand where we are in our own professional development and to define our needs and expectations regarding ongoing learning. It is worth remembering that we can be both a novice and expert at the same time in different areas of practice, dependent on how far expertise has been developed in a given area. On qualification a practitioner's skills may be less than competent in some areas despite a judgement having been made overall about his or her competence to practise. Further up the professional ladder, levels of competence may develop significantly in selected areas of practice, through a state of proficiency to a level of expertise whereby the individual will be regarded as a specialist. However, as some skills become highly developed, others may remain underdeveloped and some may fade. Competence, proficiency and expertise become intertwined as the practitioner claims a breadth of knowledge and skills but at different levels of understanding for each aspect of his or her work.

Sometimes practitioners may opt to develop expertise as a generalist and develop proficiency in a broad range of skill areas. This may arise as a result of opportunity (or lack of opportunity) for professional development in employment or because the individual has made an informed decision to develop him or herself in this way. Learning strategies can be put into place to suit the generalist or specialist, dependent on the need or desire for breadth or depth of skill development. Knowing how to learn facilitates the planning of professional development in such a way that it reflects personal needs and enhances career prospects.

Professional artistry

Becoming a competent practitioner entails learning how to become a professional artist. Fish & Twinn (1997) maintained that professional artists are those individuals who can use their own professional judgement in a creative way. They viewed a competent practitioner as a professional artist who can see frameworks and patterns rather than prescriptions and rules, and who can manage the uncertainty of professional practice. This assertion assumes that practitioners who can work with uncertainty can adapt and apply professional skills in a variety of circumstances and contexts. In this way they are equipped to practise.

The state of being a professional artist is brought about by a mode of learning in which the learner's experience is central to the learning process (Fish & Twinn, 1997). According to these authors, competence is gained through a learning process that involves experiencing, reflecting, enquiring and gaining insights. These processes need to be facilitated by skilled people. The development of competence is therefore concerned with the overall development of the practitioner who is enabled to find an approach to exploring, addressing and solving problems using principles of practice and professional judgement. In order to become a competent practitioner an individual must learn how to use experience and reflection to his or her advantage, and to learn how they may be used effectively in the future. In this way student practitioners become equipped to learn.

References

Dowie, J. & Elstein, A. (1988) *Professional Judgement – A Reader in Clinical Decision Making.* Cambridge University Press, Cambridge.

Dreyfus, H. & Dreyfus, S. (1986) *Mind over Machine: The Power of Human Intuition and Expertise in the Era of the Computer.* Blackwell, Oxford.

Dutton, R. (1995) *Clinical Reasoning in Physical Disabilities.* Williams and Wilkins, Baltimore.

Fish, D. & Twinn, S. (1997) *Quality Clinical Supervision in the Health Care Professions – Principled Approaches to Practice.* Butterworth Heinemann, Oxford.

Gratton, L. & Pearson, J. (1994) Empowering leaders: are they being developed? In *Managing Learning* (C. Mabey & P. Iles, eds). Routledge, London.

Higgs, J. (1997) Learning to make clinical decisions. In *Facilitating Learning in Clinical Settings* (L. McAllister, M. Lincoln, S. McLeod & D. Maloney, eds). Stanley Thornes, Cheltenham.

Higgs, J. & Jones, M. (1995) *Clinical Reasoning in the Health Professions.* Butterworth Heinemann, Oxford.

Chapter 7
The Adult Learner

Personal expectations and needs

Previous chapters have addressed issues relating to competence to practise and the characteristics of learning that underpin competence development and continuing professional development. This chapter sets learning into a theoretical framework of adult learning and examines ways of ensuring that effective learning takes place.

> 'Those aiming for professional qualifications or participating in updating or continuing professional development courses are individuals with personal expectations and life-plans'.

Watson (1992, p. 6) made this comment about students in the higher education system but it could be true of all individuals contemplating or participating in any continuing professional development activity. It implies that there is a purpose for the activity that has a direct bearing on each individual's personal circumstances and not just on the circumstances of their employment. It goes beyond meeting the needs of services and service users to meeting the personal needs of the learner in the widest possible sense.

Each one of us will have personal aspirations and goals for the future even though they may not all relate to our professional or career development. These affect our commitment to learning and skill development. For example, some may consider taking a break from professional practice to return to full-time study, to have a change of career or to become a full-time parent. Others may wish to travel the world. Some practitioners may be content to balance a social life with work, and just keep sufficiently abreast of the changes that affect practice to be able to maintain a professional role. Others will have a commitment to develop professionally, not just to update professional knowledge but to develop expertise and skills in order to advance in a career. Whatever the plan, an element of learning is likely to be involved. Some understanding of learning theory, most particularly of adult learning theory and styles of learning, can help to produce more effective learners and improve one's capacity to achieve personal ambitions, whatever they may be.

Adult learners

Adults engage in educational activity because of 'some innate desire for developing new skills, acquiring new knowledge, improving already assimilated competencies or sharpening powers of self-insight' (Brookfield, 1986, p. 11). This applies equally to personal interests as to professionally-oriented activities. However, it should not be forgotten that developing knowledge and skills is not just for immediate gain but is also as an investment for the future. Certainly, Longworth & Davies (1996) noted that increasingly the onus is on individuals to invest in skills for their personal growth and to develop their own potential. Part of the rationale behind this expectation is the rapidity of change in professional life and the need for individuals to develop a repertoire of competencies in order to remain skilled for employment. Developing new skills and interests can provide 'strings to the bow' in the event of unexpected changes in employment, roles or responsibilities.

Craft (1996) listed a number of personal reasons for individuals wishing to engage in continuing professional development:

- To improve job performance
- To develop professional knowledge and understanding
- For career development or promotion
- To promote job satisfaction
- To develop an enhanced view of the job
- To anticipate and prepare for change

This is unlikely to be an exhaustive list but does give some idea of the reasons why practitioners might wish to continue to learn. It supplements the list of benefits that came from continuing professional development listed in Chapter 1. Most professionals would identify with at least one of the above reasons regardless of any need that relates to service development or improvement in service quality. Although initial professional education has to be controlled and directed because it has to meet professional specifications, continuing professional development offers far more choice in the way in which individuals participate in learning activities in order to meet personal needs and expectations.

Adult learning theory

There is a theoretical side to learning that guides adults in their endeavours to develop skills and that helps facilitators of learning to approach adult education in a way that is sensitive to individuals' experiences, needs and values. Exploring the theoretical aspects of learning provides a basis for understanding how preferred learning styles and learning strategies can be used to advantage in ways that are acceptable and likely to lead to positive results. Much has been written in the past about adult learning theory. It is certainly not the intention here to expound those theories but only to show how theory can help us to understand the way in which we learn so we may become more effective learners in our endeavours to meet personal and professional goals. Not only does learning theory aid the individual, but it can also aid facilitators of learning in their approach to adult education so that it is sensitive to an individual's experiences, needs and values.

Knowles (1990) presented what he called the *foundation stones of modern adult learning theory*. These can be summarised in the following way.

(1) Adults are motivated to learn as they experience needs and interests that learning will satisfy
(2) An adult's orientation to learning is determined by, and centred on, his or her life's circumstances
(3) An adult's life experiences are the richest source of learning
(4) Adults primarily need to be self-directed in their learning activity
(5) Individual differences among people increase with age so that personal differences in the style, time, place and pace of learning must be acknowledged

If these statements are true then we can deduce that adults like to be in control of their learning so that they can choose the pace and means of addressing their learning needs. They prefer to direct their attention to matters that are meaningful and that have a purpose, are relevant and of interest to them in relation to their lives. Adults already have a wealth of experience on which to draw and new experiences will provide them with opportunities to integrate new learning with former experiences so that new insights emerge to be used in the future.

The nature of learning

Whenever we take steps to develop professionally we are engaging in learning. Learning has been considered as both a process and a product and has been variously defined by theorists over time. Yet having offered a critique of many of the definitions, Knowles (1990) concluded that learning is an 'elusive phenomenon' that seems to defy definition. The bulk of opinion, however, favours the concept of learning as a process. Knowles reminds us of some of the great teachers of the past such as Aristotle, Socrates, Plato and Cicero who commonly perceived learning to be a process of active inquiry and not just of passive acceptance of information. Little has changed in the arguments over time. Curzon (1990, p. 31) also viewed learning as a process 'of interaction as a result of which the learner gains fresh insights, so shedding or modifying previously held perceptions'. In the same way Mezirow (1991) asserted that learning is a process of interpretation of experiences and of making meaning, reinforcing the earlier claim by Combs (1971) that learning is the discovery of meaning. The meaning derived from learning experiences will be personal and different for each individual.

Jarvis (1995, p. 65), referring to concepts expounded earlier by Dewey (1916), stated that 'learning always begins with experiencing'. Throughout their lives, individuals accumulate a wide range of experiences that are stored in the memory and brought to every new or potential learning situation. These memories can influence the way in which new experiences are interpreted so making the experience both individual and personal. Learning is the process of transforming experience into knowledge, skills, attitudes, values and emotions. It can arise from both primary and secondary experiences. Primary experiences are those where individuals enter into the situation and experience at first hand. Secondary experiences tend to be those arising from communication, for example, through conversation, listening to lectures or reading books. Meaning is communicated through words and pictures. These can be expressed as learning provided that interaction has been built into the experience. As Jarvis pointed out, a great deal of everyday life is dialogue and interaction and this should not be ignored as a source of learning. The quality of learning in these situations, however, is likely to depend on the receptiveness of the learner to the potential of learning from the situation.

Experiential learning

Boud *et al.* (1993, p. 6) reiterated Dewey's proposition that experience is a 'meaningful encounter', an active engagement with the environment where the learner forms part of the total scene and makes his or her contribution to the experience. What occurs is a process of learning and what results is an outcome of learning that is unique to the individual. As Mezirow (1991) claimed, the meaning of the experience is an essential part of the experience. New learning derives from the experience and this is set into the context of existing knowledge and understanding. New experiences can provide new learning or they can prompt a reinterpretation of existing knowledge and understanding built up through previous experiences. However, Boud and his colleagues point out that while the experience of learning may be the foundation of learning itself, it does not necessarily lead to it. Active engagement in the experience and exploration of it is crucial so that experience is transformed into meaningful learning. Exploration takes place through the process of reflection which contributes to conceptual understanding (Thorpe, 1993). Unless an experience is examined and reflected upon it has no educational value (Criticos, 1993).

Boud *et al.* (1993, p. 9) defined reflection as 'those processes in which learners engage to recapture, notice and re-evaluate their experience, to work with the experience and turn it into learning'. Dialogue with other people helps the reflective process and provides other perspectives to enhance the learning that transpires. Henry (1989) suggested that learning has to be taken a stage further. She noted that the ability to apply new-found knowledge has to be part of the experiential learning process in order to complete the learning cycle that Kolb (1984) originally set out. Henry accepted that the outcomes of experiential learning for an individual can include those related to *personal development*, for example, attributes such as self-awareness and confidence, as well as those related to *competence development* such as competence in communication skills and decision making.

So what does this mean for continuing professional development? It means that professionals, as adults, already have a range of experiences on which to draw and build. Further learning can take place in all sorts of situations and from many different kinds of experiences, both in formal education and through informal interactions. Each practitioner will have a preferred way of learning that enables him or her to learn effectively from different experiences. A range of activities undertaken outside the more formal academic environment can be classified as learning experiences, provided that the participating practitioner has been active in the learning process, has derived some new insights from the experiences through reflection and engagement in the learning process, and is able to integrate the new learning into practice. Henry (1989) acknowledged the growing importance and centrality of learning from experience. She listed some experiential learning strategies. They include problem-based learning, project work, independent work with learning contracts, placements or attachments, and the recognition of prior learning experiences. These are explored later. Boud (1988) conveniently classified these as three different approaches to self-directed learning, namely:

(1) *The individual-centred approach* that focuses on individual learners and their needs which are addressed, for example, through a learning contract.
(2) *The group-centred approach* that focuses on the needs of the group but where individuals pursue their own learning needs within the context of the group, gaining support and feedback from group members and learning from their interactions.
(3) *The project-centred approach* where the learning project or task becomes the focus of attention and gives meaning to group activity, for example, in problem-based learning.

All these approaches to adult learning require the learner to be self-directed and to take responsibility for his or her own learning.

Self-directed and independent learning

According to Brookfield (1986) self-directed learning refers to the activity of acquiring skills and knowledge with a minimum of professional assistance. One of the most commonly cited definitions of self-directed learning, however, is that coined by Knowles (1975). He saw it as a process in which individuals take the initiative in diagnosing needs, designing learning experiences, locating resources and evaluating learning. He developed a self-rating instrument so that individuals could assess their own level of competence in relation to self-directed learning skills. Based on Knowles' assessment tool, the competencies required of a self-directed learner can be summarised as an ability to:

- Explain the difference between underlying assumptions about teacher-directed and self-directed learning.
- Conceptualise oneself as a non-dependent and self-directed person.
- Relate to peers and other people and see them as a resource for diagnosing needs, planning learning and for learning.
- Diagnose personal learning needs realistically with help from teachers and peers.
- Translate learning needs into achievable learning objectives.
- Identify and draw on human and material resources as appropriate for addressing different learning objectives.
- Collect and validate evidence of the accomplishment of various kinds of learning objectives.

There are key differences between teacher-directed and self-directed learning that are fundamental to the learning process. These need to be understood in terms of expectations and responsibilities of the learner. Self-directed learning requires self-management in learning, independence in the pursuit of learning and critical evaluation of the learning that has taken place.

In the process of continuing professional development, self-directed learning can be applied to two scenarios. First, where a programme of learning has been organised by someone else, the learner has to take the initiative to access resources, read widely and address the requirements of the given curriculum using the resources effectively. Second, it can apply when the initiative has to be taken first to determine learning goals and then to devise and follow a strategy for meeting them, in other words to define and fulfil learning needs, accessing and using resources as required. This would be the case if one was working to a learning contract. The second scenario could more reasonably be described as independent learning. Often the term 'independent learning' is used interchangeably with self-directed learning although the concept is different.

There is no doubt that being self-directed in learning can be difficult for the learner and can be a fairly isolating activity, requiring particular motivation and well-developed support networks. Brookfield (1986) found that independent learners needed accessible peer support and network systems. Brookfield maintained that these are essential so that learners can share experiences and measure their own development against that of other people. In this way networks of learners can act as a sounding board for each other for personal reflections, for the generation of new ideas and, as Brookfield put it, as 'resource consultants' to explore how new ideas might be taken forward and used in practice.

Brookfield (1986) argued that no act of learning is fully self-directed if it is taken to mean that the learner is so self-reliant that he or she excludes all external sources of information. As he said, it is very difficult to generate alternative ways of thinking about, and behaving in, the world entirely as a result of one's own efforts. Learners who stay within their own paradigms of thinking, feeling and behaving are limiting their opportunity to learn with and from others and to being exposed to diverse ways of thinking and acting. Self-directed learning as an adult is about learning how to change perspectives, shift paradigms and replace one way of interpreting the world with another. Self-directed learning thus expects the learner to search widely for appropriate resources and to use them effectively to support the learning process. As learning occurs, a shift in perspective becomes evident so that situations are construed differently the next time around in the light of experience.

Knowledge of the learning process and of learning approaches helps to establish the responsibilities of the learner so that expectations, particularly of other people, do not become unrealistic. Taking responsibility as a self-directed learner also enables full benefit to be gained from learning opportunities that are presented. Whether the learner chooses to engage in the learning situation will often depend on the way it is presented and whether it is compatible with the learner's preferred learning style. The approach to learning that the learner takes will ultimately reflect the quality of new learning and the ability to use new-found knowledge in different situations.

Motivation to learn will dictate the extent to which a learner engages in learning experiences. Different approaches to learning give different results. Deep learning, for example, will be longer lasting than surface learning because it involves the learner pursuing a quest for understanding new information and for integrating it into existing knowledge. Surface learning, on the other hand, is an approach that involves memorising and reproducing material at face value and at the expense of understanding. Deep learning expects active participation whereas surface learning is a much more passive activity. Approaches to learning as outlined above have been described by Boud (1988) as characteristic of the interaction between an individual and a learning task. Learning styles, on the other hand, stem from personality and from a particular leaning towards some learning tasks rather than others. This is described below.

Learning styles

Entwistle (1981) argued that fundamental differences in personality affect our styles of learning – our preferred way of thinking and obtaining knowledge. We therefore choose to learn in a particular way because it suits our personality. A learning style can be said to be a 'preference or habitual strategy used by an individual to process information for problem-solving' (Katz & Heimann, 1991). Honey and Mumford (1992) modified Kolb's (1984) original work on learning styles inventories to devise a questionnaire that can be self-administered to help individuals determine their preferred learning style. On completion of the questionnaire, an individual can see whether he or she has a dominance in one learning style or another or has a broad range of learning ability across various styles. Learners are classified as four types: activists, pragmatists, reflectors and theorists. Because they relate to personality each one of these learner types has particular traits that lead an individual to work and learn in a particular way.

It is important to note that no learning style is better than any other. It is just that knowledge of our dominant style (if we have one) helps us to learn more effectively. We will tend to choose a mode of learning with which we will feel most comfortable. This means that we select learning tasks according to the learning style that we favour. An indication of whether we have a preference for a particular style of learning, or whether we have a broad range of learning ability with no clear preference, can therefore be useful. Selecting the most favourable mode of learning that is compatible with one's learning style can optimise learning, and give the most benefit from any learning opportunity presented. In selecting preferred modes of learning, individuals will tend to reject those modes with which they feel least comfortable. Honey and Mumford described how people may use awareness of their preferred style to develop effective strategies for learning in a range of situations. Some people may purposely choose modes of learning that are less favoured just so that they can develop the ability to use alternative modes of learning. The authors explain how a repertoire of learning strategies can be expanded so that learning ability is enhanced.

Becoming an effective learner

A little knowledge of adult learning theory and strategies can help to channel learning in ways that are going to be most relevant and personally effective. It helps to understand why some learning strategies can be more effective than others and to know why learning can sometimes be ineffective. At least it is possible to do something about it if the cause is understood. Knowledge of difficulties encountered in learning helps to reassure us that sometimes, no matter how hard we try, the strategy we have adopted is not going to help our learning. Learning still requires active participation but practitioners are busy people and time is always at a premium. Refining learning techniques and skills, using knowledge of what works best and why, can help us to make the most of learning opportunities as they arise. Expanding a personal repertoire of learning strategies in order to become a more effective learner is possible (Honey & Mumford, 1992), and certainly a good idea if it will facilitate learning in new ways.

It is also worth remembering that there can be a number of other barriers to learning. These will be familiar to most practitioners but may not be recalled and applied to their own learning situation. Fatigue, stress, an environment that is not conducive to learning, poor organisation, poor concentration, poor motivation, or a lack of opportunity to practise new skills or apply new knowledge can all interfere with learning. When taking responsibility for learning we have to take responsibility for finding the optimum environment in which learning can take place. It is easy to argue that circumstances will not always be favourable and that a learning environment is hardly ever ideal but there are factors that we can control and it is possible at least to take some responsibility for making the circumstances for learning as favourable as they can be. Effective learning is at the root of continuing professional development.

References

Boud, D. (ed.) (1988) *Developing Student Autonomy in Learning*. Kogan Page, London.

Boud, D., Cohen, R. & Walker, D. (eds) (1993) *Using Experience for Learning*. The Society for Research into Higher Education and Open University Press, Buckingham.

Brookfield, S. (1986) *Understanding and Facilitating Adult Learning*. Open University Press, Milton Keynes.

Combs, A.W. (1971) Helping relationships: basic concepts for the helping professions. Allyn & Bacon, Boston. Cited in M. Knowles (1990) *Adult Learner a Neglected Species*. Gulf Publishing Company, Houston.

Craft, A. (1996) *Continuing Professional Development – A Practical Guide for Teachers and Schools*. Routledge, London.

Criticos, C. (1993) Experiential learning and social transformation for a post-apartheid learning future. In *Using Experience for Learning* (D. Boud, R. Cohen & D. Walker, eds). The Society for Research into Higher Education and Open University Press, Buckingham.

Curzon, L.B. (1990) *Teaching in Further Education – An Outline of Principles and Practice*, 4th edn. Cassell, London.

Dewey, J. (1916) Democracy and education. Cited in S. Brookfield (1986) *Understanding and Facilitating Adult Learning*. Open University Press, Milton Keynes.

Entwistle, N. (1981) *Styles of Learning and Teaching*. John Wiley & Son, London.

Henry, J. (1989) Meaning and practice in experiential learning. In *Making Sense of Experiential Learning: Diversity in Theory and Practice* (S. Warner Weil & I. McGill, eds). The Society for Research into Higher Education and Open University Press, Buckingham.

Honey, P. & Mumford, A. (1992) *The Manual of Learning Styles*. Peter Honey, Ardingly House, Maidenhead, Berks.

Jarvis, P. (1995) *Adult and Continuing Education*, 2nd edn. Routledge, London.

Katz, N. & Heimann, N. (1991) Learning styles of students and practitioners in five health professions. *The Occupational Therapy Journal of Research* **11**, 238–45.

Knowles, M. (1975) *Self-directed Learning: A Guide for Learners and Teachers*. Prentice Hall, Englewood Cliffs.

Knowles, M. (1990) *Adult Learner a Neglected Species*. Gulf Publishing Company, Houston.

Kolb, D. (1984) *Experiential Learning*. Prentice Hall, Englewood Cliffs.

Longworth, N. & Davies, W.K. (1996) *Lifelong Learning*. Kogan Page, London.

Mezirow, J. (1991) Transformative dimensions of adult learning. Cited in P. Jarvis (1995) *Adult and Continuing Education*, 2nd edn. Routledge, London.

Thorpe, M. (1993) Experiential learning at a distance. In: *Using Experience for Learning* (D. Boud, R. Cohen & D.Walker, eds). The Society for Research into Higher Education and Open University Press, Buckingham.

Watson, D. (1992) The changing shape of professional education In *Developing Professional Education* (H. Bines. & D. Watson, eds). The Society for Research into Higher Education and Open University Press, Buckingham.

Chapter 8
The Workplace as a Learning Environment

Organisational culture and policy

The organisation in which you work will have its own culture, aims and goals. These will reflect the local interpretation of the Government's agenda for health and social care. As an employee you will be expected to contribute to activities that enable the organisation to achieve these goals. The organisational culture and the policies that guide service provision and make explicit its priorities are likely to have quite an influence on the way in which you practise. It is therefore important that you gain an understanding of the policies and the rationale behind them so that you can work according to the service's expectations and needs. An organisation that encourages its staff to become aware of its business plan and to understand the service philosophy and organisational structures, and one which involves staff in policy formation and supports them in their endeavours to contribute effectively to service provision is more likely to be successful in achieving its goals. In this respect the organisation becomes a learning environment where employees can develop skills and expertise and contribute effectively to the organisation's activities. Engaging in organisational learning can thus aid your personal and professional development.

One of the activities that supports the organisation's business is the formulation of policies, procedures, priorities and protocols that underpin professional practice. It can be seen as development activity to become involved in the generation of policy that aims to seek the best outcome for service users. It may be necessary to acknowledge that sometimes the values that underpin service policies and service provision will be at variance with your own values and the value systems of your profession. Nevertheless, the overall aims of the service in which you work will consistently be to meet the needs of its users in the best possible way, and to be able to modify its practices to reflect changes in the wider environment that inevitably impact on service provision.

Organisations are forever subject to the influences of the wider environment in which they operate. External drivers of change, particularly in health and social care, tend to stem from new social policies. The interpretation of policy in relation to service provision and major changes in the strategic direction of the service can mean that staff need to acquire new skills for practice, or to learn to use existing skills differently in new contexts of practice. The employing organisation cannot therefore ignore its responsibilities to ensure that staff have the right level of skills for the job they are doing and to develop the skills of its employees when these are found to be lacking or in need of modification. The effectiveness of service provision could otherwise be adversely affected. Both you and the service in which you work thus have responsibilities with regard to continuing professional development. Engaging actively in the business of the organisation can therefore be to your mutual benefit.

Quality and change

Organisations have wide ranging obligations if the services they are to provide to the public are to be effective. Cost-effective services operated according to a set of standards, monitored for quality and improved through feedback, is the ultimate goal. If quality assurance mechanisms are to be effective, feedback from service users must indicate where modifications to service provision may be required and staff must take steps to accommodate changes that are shown to be beneficial. Employers must therefore take responsibility for ensuring that staff develop professionally so that they can adapt in response to changing circumstances. Effective organisations depend to a large extent on the quality of staff they employ, the manner in which they deploy them and the strategies used to retain and develop them. Staff development thus needs to be integral to organisational life for the maintenance of quality and the management of change. It therefore has to be resourced appropriately.

As far as staff development is concerned, it has consistently been said that responsibility for CPD rests largely with the individual. Each practitioner has to ensure that his or her practice is evaluated, that limitations in skills or gaps in knowledge are identified, and that plans are made and pursued to ensure that competence is maintained. Employers have a duty to support individuals to maintain their competence at least to a level that ensures their fitness to practise safely within the organisation. This is both a professional and organisational responsibility that minimises risk of harm to users and risk of litigation for the individual and employing authority. The aim of staff development, however, is not just to provide the minimum capacity to get by, but to ensure the highest quality of service provision for users using the resources available. This means that organisations must take steps to develop a highly skilled workforce in recognition of their responsibility to ensure that staff are competent to practise within the service, and that they remain so.

Eraut (1994) observed that new knowledge is rarely sought for the ongoing improvement of practice within an organisation; it is normally sought only where it enables individuals to cope with external demands for change. This would suggest that practitioners need to be very clear about their rationale for continuing professional development and must negotiate for CPD in order to improve their practice, and not just to maintain it at a basic level of competence. Staff development programmes initiated within the organisation and supported by personal development plans can help to ensure that employees continue to improve their effectiveness and are enabled to fulfil the organisation's changing needs and goals. Redman (1994) argued that organisations need to be committed to the ideals of development through a process of learning where everyone is involved. The only way to do this successfully is for the service environment to operate according to the principles of a learning organisation that facilitates the growth of staff and their commitment to and capacity to achieve organisational goals.

Learning organisations

The organisation is the context for service provision but it also serves as the context in which all staff activity takes place. If services are going to be effective and staff are to remain committed to their work then the culture of the organisation has to be conducive to learning and development. As Harvey-Jones (1987) pointed out, organisations will only survive if they aim to meet the needs of the staff who serve in them. Staff need to have an interest in the work that they do which must help them to grow personally. Those organisations that see themselves as learning organisations espouse a culture of learning and of working to facilitate staff and organisational development in a climate of change.

As you read through the next few paragraphs it might be worth thinking about the extent to which your employing organisation might be considered a learning organisation. It might also be worth considering what you and others might do to promote continuing professional development within your employing organisation in the light of the principles known to underpin learning organisations.

Characteristics of learning organisations

Garrett (1990) identified three characteristics of learning organisations:

- They encourage people at all levels to learn regularly and rigorously from their work.
- They have systems in place for capturing the learning and for moving staff with skills to where they are needed in the organisation.
- They value learning and use it to transform the organisation.

The culture of the learning organisation thus seems to be one of striving for improvement and for quality in service provision by valuing learning, by developing the skills of the workforce and by deploying skilled people where they can best serve the organisation's needs. It involves living in and managing a state of uncertainty where questioning and change are the norm (Dale, 1994). It means responding to learning by getting rid of outdated practice and replacing it with practice that has been shown to be more effective or relevant in today's climate. Ultimately this strategy is likely to benefit service users, the organisation and its employees, but organisational life is not just about meeting current needs, it is about evolving and growing to meet future needs.

Senge (1990) viewed a learning organisation as one that is constantly expanding its capacity to create its future. By facilitating the learning of all its members the learning organisation continuously transforms itself (Dale, 1994). Transformation is a common theme in the literature about learning organisations as it is recognised that every organisation has to adapt to environmental changes and this has to occur through the efforts of its employees. According to Pearn *et al.* (1995) a learning organisation has a strong vision of its future and part of this vision recognises the importance of learning at all levels of organisational life – at the level of the individual, at team level and in relation to the organisation's systems. It is thus important for learning and staff development to be supported at each of these levels. The capacity to learn helps the organisation to survive and thrive in an increasingly unpredictable world.

Edmonstone (1990) observed how learning organisations are likely to attract 'high learning' individuals into a culture that is mutually beneficial. The focus of the learning organisation is on the individual learning to solve work-related problems in the workplace, thus enabling both the organisation and its employees to evolve and grow through their own efforts. Staff development, as an ongoing process, enables the organisation to prepare for and work with change but the organisation will only learn if its individual members learn and bring about change (Swieringa & Wierdsma, 1992). The fact is, change is a certainty and knowledge decay or knowledge obsolescence is a problem because of the pace of change. The challenge is to be able to develop competent individuals who have the capacity to act with confidence, insight, skill and flexibility in a constantly changing world (Henry, 1989).

Given the climate today and the uncertainty of employment, Waterman *et al.* (1994) suggested that staff should demand education, training and development as a right. Certainly, Dimond (1997) suggested that bargaining facilities should be used by staff to ensure that provision is made in their contracts for paid study leave, secondment and other forms of post-registration education and training. Whilst it may be the responsibility of individuals to manage their own career, the organisation has a responsibility to provide the tools for learning and for developing the skills of the workforce. A workforce that comprises individuals who can relate to change, who are prepared to update skills and develop multiple skills in anticipation of change, becomes more flexible and more able to move across functional boundaries (Waterman *et al.*, 1994). A learning organisation that invests in its staff is likely to be one that attracts and retains motivated individuals who will strive for effectiveness in their work and enable the organisation to flourish.

Investing in people

One of the characteristics of a learning organisation is that it invests in its workforce. A national quality initiative known as 'Investors in People' was developed by the Training and Enterprise Council to promote education and training within organisations. Those who work on it are deemed to be taking steps towards becoming a learning organisation (Craft, 1996). Employers are invited to work towards achieving stringent, nationally set standards that are based on four management principles:

(1) A public commitment from the top to develop all employees to achieve the business' objectives.
(2) A regular review of all employees' training and development needs.
(3) Action to train and develop individuals on recruitment and throughout their employment by the organisation.
(4) An evaluation of the investment in training and development to assess achievement and improve future effectiveness.

To be recognised for the award of Investor in People, an organisation has to show its plans for the achievement of the standards and to provide a portfolio of evidence that the standards have been achieved (Redman, 1994). The organisation is assessed by independent assessors who examine policy documents, procedures and records and explore employees' experiences and understanding of the training policy and practice (Dale, 1994).

The Investors in People initiative recognises organisations whose policies and practices demonstrate a commitment to staff for their training and development. Those who work towards achieving the requirements of the Investors in People award 'are conscious of the need to show both to their own staff and to the outside world their commitment to quality' (Redman, 1994, p. 157). The hope is that organisations will integrate training and development into their business planning and so see it as a long-term investment to improve performance and achieve corporate objectives (Keep, 1993).

The message is clear for health practitioners. Continuing professional development is more likely to be supported in environments that strive for effectiveness by encouraging and supporting learning. Learning in the workplace is one way of developing skills that will benefit the service but it should also be remembered that learning beyond the workplace, through higher education, is likely to be equally, and sometimes more, beneficial to the organisation and service users. However, the links between service development and growth have sometimes to be made explicit before this kind of education is supported by managers.

Learning managers

Managers are the people who ensure that the staff for whom they are responsible operate according to the goals and policies of the organisation and use their skills to achieve the most effective outcome for service users. Whether or not the service is to be seen as a learning organisation, managers have a duty to support staff in their endeavours to work to the highest possible standards, fulfil service obligations and to promote and cooperate with service developments. As Dale (1994, p. 32) stated rather bluntly, 'being a developmental manager requires determination, commitment, effort and belief. Being a contra-developmental manager is easy. You expect nothing, give nothing and get nothing' in return. It is difficult to imagine that any manager in the health and social care professions would be unsupportive of staff and their development. This would be contrary to the principles of good practice and to the ethical code of their profession. Clearly, managers should have an overall concern for the personal development of staff and for providing the learning opportunities that are necessary both for personal growth and for organisational effectiveness (Mumford, 1994).

In order to influence the quality of service provision, managers have to take responsibility for nurturing staff and for providing a facilitative environment in which they can work, learn and develop. According to Barnett & Kemp (1994), an effective learning environment is one where staff feel supported. It is also one that has a forward looking approach, where practice is based on research and where there is an awareness of professional developments. The expansion of knowledge about health care is so rapid that there has to be easy access to new material so that staff can keep up with the changes. However, the trend has been for managers to only support staff education where the natural benefits for the service can be demonstrated. This is hardly surprising in a time of budget constraints. Clearly, safe practice has to be a priority, so training in the use of new technology and equipment, updates in health and safety requirements and developmental activity to support essential changes in service provision have to be the priority. Even if education and training is provided in-house and free of charge, there is still a notional cost associated with the release of staff and their loss from active duty with service users.

Staff seeking support for wider career development are likely to find that managers are reluctant to divert scarce resources to this cause. Supporting staff in career development initiatives can prove to be a double-edged sword. On the one hand managers may need to support staff in career development initiatives as part of their staff retention strategy. On the other hand, supporting staff to undertake education programmes for career development may lead to them seeking employment elsewhere because new opportunities become available for them to use the new-found knowledge and skills. For this reason, career development activity that has no direct benefit for the service may only be partially funded (with the staff member being asked to contribute financially to his or her professional development) or not funded at all. Time off to undertake a programme of higher education may not be granted. It is clearly up to individual employees to make a case that any programme of professional development that they wish to undertake will be of direct benefit to the service and its users.

Learning opportunities

However much it is suggested that individuals should take responsibility for their own learning, the impetus to do this can be thwarted in an environment that does not support learning and professional development. Both employers and employees need to work collaboratively:

- To promote learning within the organisation as an integral component of service delivery
- To see and seize learning opportunities as they arise
- To seek and develop learning opportunities where there are none
- To take full advantage of the learning opportunities on offer
- To support staff as they engage in learning initiatives
- To ensure that staff review the learning that has taken place, identify learning outcomes and disseminate relevant information to others
- To relate new knowledge and skills to the provision of services, with a view to improving their effectiveness

There are many opportunities for learning within an organisation but often they go unrecognised. Learning opportunities can also be created by using the environment as a resource through which to achieve learning goals.

Learning resources

If we accept that learning both for personal growth and organisational development is a desirable objective then the resources for this to happen need to be made available. If organisations cannot meet their aims without well-qualified staff then staff development and the investment in staff as a resource have to be high on the agenda. Health and social care organisations are as much concerned with change as any other organisation. Even though profit margins may not be indicators of success, the need to invest in staff development remains crucial to the organisation's business.

Ways of supporting staff include the provision of a variety of resources that individuals can tap into according to interest or need. Library and reference material is essential but books, journals, research and reference papers do need to be current and readily accessible to all staff. In-service programmes, both uniprofessional and multiprofessional, and development programmes that include opportunities for learning in established teams, provide opportunities for staff to meet, share ideas and learn with and from each other.

Work-based learning is currently being advocated in Government policies. Funds are now available from local Education and Training Consortia to support the post-qualifying continuing professional development of health care professionals, particularly where development needs coincide with national training priorities. Applications can be made for funds to support work-based learning and for shared learning initiatives across professions and agencies. The professions allied to medicine should take advantage of these resources wherever possible to support post-qualifying education, training and professional development at local level. Formal learning and informal networking do much for morale, as well as for developing staff. Mentors to whom individual staff members have access can also provide individual staff with support and guidance to facilitate their learning and career development. Setting time aside for meeting with mentors and/or with peers, for discussion relating to professional development, has to be beneficial.

Learning in the workplace

Much has been written about the facilitation of learning in the academic environment and about the learning that students of the health and social care professions undertake in fieldwork or clinical education. In both of these situations, the learning is structured by the programme curriculum. Literature about learning in the workplace for practitioners who have completed pre-registration education and want to pursue continuing professional development tends to be less accessible. Practitioners have to recognise their learning needs, identify learning opportunities and be self-directed in their learning activity. The motivation to learn has to be at least as strong, if not stronger, than for learning in an academic setting. Support for the search for new knowledge and understanding is important, but not always available. The means to validate learning in the workplace are hard to find. Many individuals need guidance on how to learn and how to use different learning strategies, on how to identify and capitalise on learning opportunities, and in the interpretation of new knowledge and its application to practice.

Work-based learning may be high on the Government's agenda, but it is not necessarily an easy option. In the academic environment an infrastructure exists to support learning but in the workplace it tends to be less clearly defined and under-resourced. This places enormous responsibility on an individual who may not be adept at managing personal learning. A high level of motivation is essential, particularly if learning outcomes are expected to relate more to the organisation's needs than to those of the individual. There may be no achievements in terms of credit or named award for the individual, just the capacity to be more effective in the workplace. Structured programmes of learning in the workplace are preferable to unstructured ones, but there also needs to be some personal incentive for participating in the learning programme. In order to promote effective work-based learning, it is essential for organisations to establish the infrastructure to support it, and this includes well-developed links with Institutes of Higher Education. Collaboration between service and academic staff in projects and research at service level can strengthen partnerships and provide opportunities for staff in both organisations to develop and demonstrate enhanced skills.

Occupational standards

The National Occupational Standards for Professional Activity in Health Promotion and Care (Care Sector Consortium, 1997) were established as a conceptual framework for working effectively in practice. The standards serve as benchmarks relating to performance, and its improvement, by acting as specifications of good practice. The Occupational Standards purport to describe performance in terms of what *should* happen (rather than what *does* happen) and the knowledge, understanding and skills that individuals are likely to need in order to meet the expectations of employment (Mitchell, 1998). They are based on a Job Competence Model which embraces four key aspects of all work roles (Mansfield & Mitchell, 1996):

(1) The technical expectations
(2) The ability to work with uncertainty
(3) The ability to manage different and sometimes conflicting demands of the work role
(4) The ability to manage and work within environmental constraints

Occupational Standards for post-qualifying practice were developed cooperatively with professional bodies representing most of the professions allied to medicine. The 'PAMs' project had three main themes:

(1) Managing care services and facilities
(2) Managing disability and change
(3) Assessment and care planning

The National Occupational Standards originally underpinned the National Vocational Qualifications structure, now much-used by health and social care support workers. They were never intended to underpin the development of professional qualifications (Harvey, 1998) but specified the expected minimum level of performance of professionals one year after qualification. Cheesman (1998) suggested that the standards fit well into the Government's agenda of service quality enhancement, ensuring organisational fitness and a workforce capable of responding to change. The National Occupational Standards are thus intended to provide a structure for learning to practise effectively in the workplace, in order to make a constructive contribution to service delivery and to improve the care given to service users. If standards are further developed and validated by both professional and statutory regulatory bodies they may become the acknowledged benchmarks for assessing continued competence in the workplace (Powell, 1999).

In summary, there seems to be a clear rationale for the education, training and further development of staff in the workplace. Services need to be effective in what they do so there is a need at least to maintain and, where possible, to improve the quality of service provision via the development of the workforce. Clinical governance is a requirement and evidence-based practice is being demanded as part of the drive for service efficiency and effectiveness. There is also a need for organisations to be able to adapt to change and to bring about change as circumstances demand. Organisations that work to the principles of a learning organisation, investing in the workforce, are more likely to demonstrate quality in service provision and more able to respond promptly to changes arising from the internal or external environment than those that do not. Both sets of circumstances necessarily require staff to develop, draw on and use different skills, and to use existing skills differently, as the need arises. If organisations are to survive, facilities within the workplace for the education, training and development of staff must be in place.

References

Barnett, D. & Kemp, N. (1994) *The A-Z of Applied Quality for Clinical Managers in Hospitals.* Chapman & Hall, London.

Care Sector Consortium (1997) *National Occupational Standards for Professional Activity in Health Promotion and Care: Foundations and Context.* HMSO, London.

Cheesman, G. (1998) The current policy context for occupational standards. *Professional Development News*, Special Issue, **Autumn**, pp 6–7.

Craft, A. (1996) *Continuing Professional Development A Practical Guide for Teachers and Schools.* Routledge, London.

Dale, M. (1994) Learning organizations. In *Managing Learning.* (C. Mabey & P. Iles, eds). Routledge, London.

Dimond, B. (1997) *Legal Aspects of Occupational Therapy.* Blackwell Science, Oxford.

Edmonstone, J. (1990) What price the learning organisation in the public sector? In *Self-development in Organisations* (M. Pedlar, J. Burgoyne, T. Boydell & G. Welshman, eds). McGraw-Hill, London.

Eraut, M. (1994) *Developing Professional Knowledge and Competence.* The Falmer Press, London.

Garrett, B. (1990) Creating a learning organisation: a guide to leadership, learning and development. Cited in M. Pearn, C. Roderick & C. Mulrooney (1995) *Learning Organisations in Practice.* McGraw-Hill, Maidenhead.

Harvey, T. (1998) National occupational standards for professional activity in health promotion and care – the contribution of the PAMs. *Professional Development News*, Special Issue, **Autumn**, p 5.

Harvey-Jones, J. (1987) *Making it Happen.* Guild Publishing, London.

Henry, J. (1989) Meaning and practice in experiential learning. In *Making Sense of Experiential Learning* (S. Warner Weil & I. McGill, eds). The Society for Research in Higher Education and Open University Press, Buckingham.

Keep, E. (1993) Missing, presumed skilled: training policy in the UK. In *Adult Learners, Education and Training.* (R. Edwards, S. Sieminski & D. Zeldin, eds). Routledge, London.

Mansfield, B. & Mitchell, L. (1996) *Towards a Competent Workforce.* Gower Press, London.

Mitchell, L. (1998) Competence and the development of occupational standards. *Professional Development News*, Special Issue, **Autumn**, pp 2–3.

Mumford, A. (1994) Individual and organizational learning: the pursuit of change. In *Managing Learning* (C. Mabey & P. Iles, eds). Routledge, London.

Pearn, M., Roderick, C. & Mulrooney, C. (1995) *Learning Organisations in Practice.* McGraw Hill, Maidenhead.

Powell, A. (1999) Assuring the Quality of Health Care Education and Training. Unpublished Interim Report to the Department of Health, Leeds.

Redman, W. (1994) *Portfolios for Development: A Guide for Trainers and Managers*. Kogan Page, London.

Senge, P. (1990) The fifth discipline – the art and practice of the learning organisation. Cited in M. Pearn, C. Roderick, & C. Mulrooney (1995) *Learning Organisations in Practice*. McGraw Hill, Maidenhead.

Swieringa, J. & Wierdsma, A. (1992) *Becoming a Learning Organisation – Beyond the Learning Curve*. Addison-Wesley, Wokingham.

Waterman, R.H. Jr., Waterman, J.A. & Collard, B.A. (1994) Towards a career-resilient workforce. Cited in P. Raggatt, R. Edwards & N. Small (eds) (1996) *The Learning Society: Challenges and Trends*. Routledge, London.

Chapter 9
Learning Opportunities and Strategies

Setting an agenda for your learning

Learning in some form or other will take place throughout your career. At times you will engage in learning that someone else has organised for you and where someone else has set the agenda for your education. At other times, you will have to set your own learning agenda and plan learning opportunities for yourself. For example, your initial qualifying programme had to meet the professional and legal requirements for state registration and the academic requirements for the educational award. It was structured in a particular way to fulfil these obligations. Your induction programme at the start of a new job would have included learning about policies and procedures regarding health and safety and ways of working within the organisation. Any rotation scheme that you completed would have enhanced learning about different aspects of the job in a formalised way. An action plan established as part of a performance review will have set out the learning and development activities that you agreed to undertake within a given timescale and before the next review. These activities are intended to benefit both you as an employee, and the organisation within which you work. The key feature of all these programmes is that there is a known structure within which you work and learn. The key difference between this organised learning and the continuing professional development that you initiate is that there may be no clear structure for the latter. Each person has to set a personal learning agenda and the timeframe within which it occurs, and then to put into place the strategies that will promote the learning process.

Clearly, if you are going to set and meet your own agenda for learning you will need to consider how you will do it. Establishing a plan for your own continuing learning and professional development can seem daunting at first until you realise that many of the skills and abilities that you need will have been developed during your qualifying education. Throughout your professional education you are likely to have experienced a range of learning and assessment processes that can be drawn on to develop your post-qualification learning. Learning can take place through structured educational programmes, such as in-service programmes arranged at work, through accredited Higher Education programmes, or through self-study or other programmes accredited by a professional body. Learning can also occur as work-based learning using many different kinds of experience to underpin the learning process. Whatever the strategy for continuing professional development, learning has to be self-initiated and often self-directed.

Becoming self-directed in learning

In Chapter 7 the competencies of a self-directed learner were outlined. Other literature such as Ferrier *et al.* (1988) and Taylor, (1997) would suggest that self-directed learning behaviour can be summarised as:

- Recognising your personal educational needs and the need for new learning
- Setting your own learning objectives or goals
- Selecting appropriate learning resources
- Defining relevant questions for study
- Accessing relevant information
- Testing your depth of understanding of what has been learned
- Evaluating your progress against learning objectives or goals

Recognising and assessing your personal education needs and setting goals will be tasks that you will need to do fairly regularly, for example, when you need to update your knowledge of technology, practice or policy in your current employment, when contemplating or undertaking a career move, or, more formally, when you prepare your personal development plan. Learning goals can be for the short term or long term. Short-term ones are more likely to relate to maintenance of competence to do your current job, and manage changes associated with it. Longer term goals may relate more to your personal interests and ambitions as you plan your future career within or beyond your current employing organisation. Short- and long-term learning goals may thus be worked on simultaneously.

When you have established some goals it is worth thinking very broadly about the resources that you might have at your disposal and quite carefully about how you select the specific resources that will help you to meet your learning needs. It is also worth identifying resources to which you readily have access and those to which you might have access on request. Resources can be both human and physical. They include organised programmes of study (internal or external to your employing organisation) books, articles and other library resources, organisational policies, procedures and reports, or even notes kept from study days or conferences you have previously attended. You need to make sure that the information is current. The pace of change can be rapid and references become out of date very quickly. You, yourself, and your peers are resources that are available to you. Your mentor, line manager and team members from other professions may also support you in your endeavours. You need to be selective and choose resources that will best satisfy your needs and help you to achieve your identified learning goals.

The ability to self-evaluate, to measure the progress of your learning, is necessary but it may not be something that comes particularly easy to you. It does not, however, have to be done on your own. You may take responsibility for collecting the information but you are likely to have access to other people who can help you to assess your learning progress. Discussion with different people and comments from a variety of sources should help you to make the judgements that you need about your learning progress.

Learning strategies

It is useful to remember that some of the experiential learning, teaching and assessment strategies that are currently used in qualifying programmes in Higher Education can be drawn on for continuing professional development. As Henry (1989) noted, experiential learning strategies include:

- Problem-based learning
- Project work
- Independent learning through contracts
- Placements/attachments/secondments
- Recognition of prior learning experiences

Problem-based learning

Problem-based learning has been introduced into the curricula of many programmes leading to a qualification in the health professions as a way of enabling students to develop the required reasoning skills and critical thinking needed for practice. The aim of any professional education is to prepare individuals for their role as practitioners who need to be resourceful and self-directed in their learning and in their practice. Problem-based learning has been promoted as one strategy that encourages the development of these qualities and enables individuals to learn to work collaboratively in teams to address issues related to the provision of health care.

Henry (1989) summarised the process of problem-based learning as starting with a problem, exploring it, generating possible solutions, selecting one, implementing it and revising it as necessary. It comprises design processes, experience, evaluation and feedback, and offers the opportunity for involvement in decision-making. Problem-based learning thus helps to develop 'process knowledge', such as knowing where to find, and how to use, resources effectively, knowing how to reason, make judgements and to solve problems faced in practice (Taylor, 1997). Barnett (1997) suggested that process knowledge is more important than pure knowledge, as pure knowledge may be insufficient for survival in a world of change.

In a professional qualifying programme, the situations that students explore during problem-based learning are similar to those that will be encountered later in professional life. They may be real or simulated situations. Learners interact, engage in dialogue and discussion, and share relevant knowledge and experience to address issues (Margetson, 1994). Individuals thus take responsibility for their learning, seeking out and assembling their own evidence and formulating their own deductions and decisions about the problems set (Barnett, 1994). Students contribute individually but take collective responsibility for addressing problems. Problem-based learning thus allows for ownership of learning and fosters independence of inquiry.

Problem-based learning aims to develop problem-solving, communication and other learning skills that will enable individuals to become autonomous, lifelong learners in the rapidly changing environment in which they live (Higgs, 1988). Students *learn how to learn* (Margetson, 1994) and how to take responsibility for their learning, so that learning skills can be drawn on when they are needed throughout their professional career. Problem-based learning is also an appropriate approach for team learning where all members can contribute to solving a problem relevant to their natural work environment. They can pool their resources and consider issues from a range of different professional perspectives to come up with a collective proposal and to plan a way forward.

This overview of problem-based learning simplifies what is essentially a very sophisticated strategy for learning and teaching. Readers should consult specialist texts for more details. What is important, however, is that problem-based learning is a strategy for learning that can continue beyond qualifying education to enable practitioners to address practice issues with colleagues. Problem-based learning demands a high degree of self-direction but is clearly an important process, not only for dealing with the current complexities of practice but also for preparing for the future through continuing professional development.

It is not difficult to see how the concept of problem-based learning used at pre-qualifying level is a useful concept that can guide ongoing post-qualification learning. If you enjoy working as a team member, seeking out and sharing knowledge about common issues, and particularly if you have been introduced to this approach to learning earlier in preparation for your career, then the same principles can be applied later for continuing professional development. Working in a group or team provides a framework, however loose, within which you can work and learn collaboratively and provides the momentum for learning and for keeping learning on track.

Project work

Problem-based learning is one form of 'project work' that is often, but not exclusively, used for facilitating learning about clinical cases and their management. But there are different types of projects that also draw on self-directed learning skills and that can also be classified as experiential learning.

Young (1996, p. 14) described a project as 'a collection of linked activities carried out in an organised manner with a clearly defined start point and end point to achieve some specific results'. In the academic setting, a project would have a clear remit where a student might be expected to explore a hypothetical or real-life situation, drawing on various sources of data and using them to support arguments or proposals for change. If carried out in the workplace, an individual or team would be given a remit for a project that would aim to satisfy the current strategic needs of the organisation. The outcome would be an agenda for achieving change within the service in a clearly structured way. Project work carried out in the workplace therefore presents a learning opportunity for the employee whilst at the same time producing clear results for the employing organisation. So there are benefits for both. A project is time-limited and success depends on taking a disciplined approach to achieving the results required. As Young pointed out, it provides a unique opportunity to learn new skills and a valuable way of improving performance.

Using project work as a strategy for learning would involve:

- Defining the tasks in terms of goals to be achieved in the workplace
- Establishing the parameters of the task
- Identifying the resources that are necessary to complete it
- Setting an agenda for action
- Establishing the timeframe within which the activity must be complete

The needs of all the stakeholders have to be taken into consideration. The project would normally be managed by a project manager or supervisor who allocates work and retains an overview of how resources are being used, takes responsibility for keeping the project on track and on time, and facilitates the resolution of problems that arise. The project manager generally acts as a 'sounding board' for matters arising during the project. Small projects can be carried out entirely by one individual as a learning experience and way of achieving a service-related goal. Alternatively, individuals from the service can be nominated for membership of a larger team to work collaboratively on a project or programme of service development.

Learning can derive from either being the project supervisor or manager or from being a member of a project group. As a project supervisor you are likely to be involved in discussions about the resolution of various problems and concerns as they arise. As mentioned above, you will have overall responsibility for the operational management of the project, co-ordinating the activity and keeping it on schedule. As a member of a project group, you might be a member of one of a number of disciplines or professions represented where there is an opportunity to learn from each other by working together. You may have to negotiate the time you can spend on the project. You will need to learn to integrate project work into your normal duties unless you are seconded full time. You will thus develop the ability to work to tight schedules and deadlines. As you can imagine, project work can provide an opportunity for you to learn something about yourself and your ability to manage the different elements of your workload within the time you have available. To complete the project you may be required to research and process information and use it in new ways. You may have to define options for problem resolution and appraise options for their costs and benefits. Skills of inquiry, analysis and self-management will almost certainly be developed in the process.

You may be elected to be a member of a project group because you have some special knowledge, skills or experience that can contribute to the work. You may use your knowledge and skills in new ways, or adapt your skills to suit the project, so adding to your expertise. You are likely to experience the dynamics of working with the team, coming into contact with people with a different range of expertise and perspectives to your own, and you can learn from them. The project may take you into different environments that also become new contexts for learning. You may have to present your contribution to the team verbally or in writing, or you may have to devise a strategy for implementing the project and this may mean that you need to market your plan to colleagues. All the different facets of learning though project work can be evaluated and recorded in a portfolio as part of the process of continuing professional development.

In work too, project management is an experiential learning strategy that can be applied to many situations where change is perceived to be needed. Work-based activity could therefore be redefined in terms of projects to be completed so that the process of their completion becomes learning that can be recognised as continuing professional development.

Action learning in project work

Action learning is about helping people learn from their day-to-day practice (Margerison, 1994, p. 109) through sharing and gaining an understanding of other people's situation. According to Margerison, action learning helps individuals to:

- Learn from experience
- Share concerns and experiences constructively with others
- Use learning from shared experiences to further the project
- Review actions taken and lessons learned

All action learning is centred around a project that is carried out as a partnership. Those who are working on the project, typically known as a 'set', come together to share problems and concerns and to learn from and support each other in undertaking the part of the work for which each has responsibility. As Margerison (1994) pointed out, the essence of action learning is that it starts with a statement of what you are trying to change in the future. It then comes back to the present and the past to identify what has to be done and what is known. It is one way of integrating both the task and the learning to bring about organisational change (Mumford, 1994).

Research as project work

Projects that are undertaken through a process of rigorous, systematic study or scientific inquiry may be referred to as research but the same principles of project work apply. A study may be carried out independently by an individual or collaboratively by a team of researchers. It may have to be completed within a given timescale and may have to address issues related to service delivery. It will not necessarily result in some organisational change but may indicate where change is needed.

Research has variously been defined as 'a course of critical study' or as 'a diligent inquiry or examination of data, reports and observations in search of facts and principles' (Drummond, 1996). Payton (1994, p. 1) referred to it simply as 'a systematic search for reliable knowledge' and Bailey (1991, p. 1) as 'the systematic investigation of a problem, issue or question'. The research project is most often undertaken using pre-defined methodology that has been carefully selected to fulfil the aims of the research and to minimise bias. Data is collected and analysed systematically. An interpretation of the data is offered. A discussion puts the findings into a theoretical context and draws conclusions based on evidence from the data. Research therefore tends to be more formalised and follows a particular pattern. It means being orderly, considered, scholarly and scientific about the work in order to validate the study. It is underpinned by principles that include (Edwards & Talbot, 1994):

- Critically appraising the problem within the current contexts of knowledge, policy and political frameworks
- Clarifying the real issues to be addressed
- Using the best evidence available
- Presenting an analysis that goes beyond description
- Offering interpretations that relate the here and now to the past and future
- Presenting a report based on the format of introduction, rationale for the study, aims, literature review, method, findings, discussion, conclusion and recommendations

Engaging in research projects and using research skills for systematic inquiry can help to provide evidence for practice and the means to justify work undertaken. It can be one of the most challenging, yet rewarding, means of learning that demands a critical and thorough approach to seeking new knowledge and to developing insights about aspects of practice.

Research has been part of the language of therapists for quite a time now, but evidence that therapists engage in research routinely as part of their practice is scant. Dowie (1994) suggested that the gap stems from inadequacies in communication. Researchers do not communicate their findings in a way that can be interpreted and applied by practitioners. Practitioners who do not have a formal grounding in research language would then seem to be disadvantaged. The consequence is that evidence emerging from research is not being used to underpin practice. Despite research being promoted as one of the activities that gives a profession credibility, researchers in the health professions are still few and far between. However, it is not necessary for everyone to be a researcher but clearly some awareness of the research process and, as Kitchen (1997) recommended, research literacy, are essential for all health professionals. There is now a minimum expectation that each practitioner can make judgements about research and locate and use evidence of research in practice.

Eakin (1997) described three possible levels of involvement in research activity, categorising practitioners as:

- Those who are research consumers (all practitioners)
- Those who are research participants (a substantial number of practitioners)
- Those who are proactive researchers (a limited number of practitioners)

There is therefore scope for each practitioner to contribute to the profession's research agenda in some way and to use the learning that emerges from the activity associated with it as evidence of continuing professional development. Collaborative work with known researchers, such as university staff, is one way of developing research skills and using them to explore a relevant work-related issue.

Evidence-based practice

Evidence-based health care has been defined as taking place when decisions that affect the care of patients are taken with due weight being given to all valid and relevant information (Hicks, 1997). It draws on the principle of using the best available evidence (and accommodating a service user's particular circumstances and personal preferences) to inform decision-making in practice and ultimately to improve the quality of clinical judgements (Rosenberg & Donald, 1995). As with evidence-based medicine, it is a process that involves systematically finding, appraising and using contemporaneous research findings as the basis for clinical decisions (Rosenberg & Donald, 1995. p. 1122). It does not automatically dictate the way that care has to be provided, it just provides the factual basis on which practitioners can make decisions.

Evidence-based practice, like research, is a systematic process and has six key steps that can be summarised as:

(1) Identifying practice-related questions that can be explored through the acquisition of data.
(2) Tracking down relevant literature from the most appropriate sources.
(3) Reviewing and critically evaluating literature for research that is valid, reliable and useful.
(4) Evaluating one's own practice in the light of the evidence emerging from the literature.
(5) Applying useful, good quality research findings to practice.
(6) Re-evaluating practice in the light of actions taken.

It is important to note that evidence-based practice is intended to build upon evidence gained from good clinical skills and sound clinical experience as this informs current *best practice*. It is not a recipe for practice but an approach that promotes the considered use of current *best evidence* in making decisions about the care of individual service users. It thus supports sound decision-making, ensures effective use of resources and results in the best possible outcomes for service users.

The one thing to reinforce is that evidence-based practice is not the same thing as research, although some of the knowledge and skills useful for carrying out research are also useful for evidence-based practice. Evidence-based practice requires individuals to have the skills to seek out research that has already been done, and then to interpret and judge the findings in relation to current practice and to introduce changes to their own practice where this seems appropriate. It should then be possible to offer a rationale for practice, based on the available evidence.

Neither evidence-based practice activity nor research activity has to be undertaken alone or in isolation. Much more learning can ensue if the activity is undertaken collaboratively with a colleague or team members. The work can be shared out and the discussions that follow can generate more ideas and new insights about practice than might be possible alone. Comparative work can be undertaken across services. Pilot schemes can be implemented and collectively evaluated before major or permanent changes are made in practice. As far as evidence-based practice is concerned, each member of the group or team can take responsibility for finding out about an aspect of practice. Subsequent discussion can lead to debates about different possibilities for action, the relative merits of each option and the possible consequences of taking a new approach. Decision-making is collective and gives shared ownership of the project. Each contributing member will be able to record some aspect of the process in relation to continuing professional development.

Why base practice on evidence?

Delivering services based on accurate and current information about practice is the essence of evidence-based practice. Whether this happens will depend on how well individual practitioners have developed the relevant professional skills to implement it. It could be suggested that new skills are needed for this to happen, but it may be that known skills already used in professional practice can be used but applied in a different way.

The pace of change in technology and techniques used in health care means that keeping up to date is a necessary, but time-consuming, activity if practice is to continue to be accurate and current. In addition, the changing expectations of the public in relation to effective health care and a greater willingness to seek redress when expectations are not fulfilled also provide the impetus for practitioners to take steps towards evidence-based practice. In the past, decisions were based on values and 'custom and practice', but now a more scientific approach is needed to provide the credibility of evidence for decision-making. Developing the skills to move away from opinion-based practice towards evidence-based practice is therefore essential (Gray, 1997).

The reasons presented above for requiring evidence-based practice are externally generated. While they are valid in themselves, it is important to recognise that a commitment of time is needed to seek evidence of best practice. The personal benefits of developing and using skills in support of evidence-based practice are not insignificant. The process can not only enhance professional skills and professional practice, but it can also provide the necessary evidence of continuing professional development (Alsop, 1997). Engaging in various research-related activities demonstrates that an individual has an enquiring mind and is questioning practice, is taking time to reflect on practice, and is hopefully developing new insights into practice. Seeking out new perspectives on practice, evaluating evidence, discriminating between the different arguments and making decisions about relevance to practice are versatile skills. It is therefore worth making the effort to develop these skills as a personal investment for the future.

Promoting a culture of evidence-based practice and research

The only way in which research data will consistently be used to inform practice is when exploring the evidence becomes second nature to practitioners and when evidence-based practice is totally embedded in clinical work. The integration of clinical and evidence-based practice, where the process of inquiry forms a normal part of care management, should allow the best service to be provided to users. This means developing a practice culture where it is acceptable as part of everyday practice to:

- Evaluate and question practice
- Explore alternative approaches to practice and present them for critical review
- Debate different approaches to practice for their potential merits
- Make judgements about the relevance of the evidence in the context of practice
- Introduce different approaches, monitor and evaluate them

These activities are not fixed in time but form part of an ongoing process that supports quality improvement in practice. It is essential, therefore, that managers as well as clinicians take responsibility for bringing research into practice. As the Chartered Society of Physiotherapy (1996) pointed out, managers have a vital role to play in creating an environment that is conducive to, and supportive of, research and evaluation in practice. Research and evaluation skills need to be valued alongside clinical skills to the extent that professional education, both pre- and post-registration, embraces the development of all the necessary skills to support evidence-based practice. In addition, practitioners who are willing and able, not just to use evidence in support of practice but also to generate evidence for practice through research, need to be supported. This means introducing research to the clinical role and balancing caseload activity with research activity in order to reap the rewards that research can bring.

Undertaking more formal activity in order to make a contribution to evidence-based health care demands a commitment from both employer and employee and an agreed plan for developing necessary skills. Some of the time to engage in these activities, which can have major benefits for the service and its users, ought to be allocated within working hours and financial resources allocated to enable the Government's agenda for evidence-based decision making to be addressed.

The main purpose here is not, however, to explain how to develop evidence-based practice. Other books offer more detailed guidance, for example Gray (1997) and Taylor (1999). The purpose is to note that professional activity related to research and evidence-based practice can and should be recorded as continuing professional development. Any one of the stages of the research process listed at the beginning of the chapter can generate activity that can be classified as CPD. Taking active steps to review and evaluate evidence of good practice or to generate new knowledge to underpin practice through research will thus be of benefit in two different, but complementary, ways. It provides evidence both of continuing professional development and of effective health care delivery.

Starting the process of inquiry

Questioning practice constructively and systematically can lead to different perspectives on and new insights about practice. This is integral to professional development. Having an open mind, being perceptive of the need for change and being receptive of new ideas are all qualities that facilitate personal learning and professional development. Learning by questioning practice thus contributes to continuing professional development.

Seeking the evidence base for practice involves questioning what currently happens in practice and what other people have done in similar situations. Evidence-based practice applies to all facets of health care delivery, including the management and education components and not just to clinical work. Evidence-based practice is about doing things right and about doing the right things, but it is also about doing things differently when there is sound evidence for change. This can mean dropping practices that custom and tradition have previously reinforced. The aim of questioning is to consider whether outcomes could be different if a different approach were to be used to deliver health care. For example, is it possible to use another approach to:

- achieve the same results more quickly or more cheaply with no long-term differences or detrimental effects?
- improve performance or quality of life?
- reduce unwanted factors?
- increase flexibility in service provision?

Any of these new outcomes may be possible by choosing a new approach backed by evidence that there are no major disadvantages to the change. Evidence-based practice requires practitioners to believe that lessons can be learned from the practice of other people. This means accepting that it is natural to enquire about what others have done and to examine critically and systematically what they do in practice, and about what they have found and recorded. *Ad hoc* comments about practice often provide the starting point for a systematic inquiry to find the evidence for practice. For example, a question may arise informally about why a particular intervention worked well for one person but not for another. Such questions may be generated through independent reflection on practice or through conversations with other people. The first step in being able to use evidence-based practice is to question practice itself.

Some of the questions that might be asked about a particular aspect of practice are as follows:

- Why do I do that?
- Do I have to do it? Could a support worker do it as successfully as me?
- Given the opportunity, do I always do it? When I don't do it is the result the same or different?
- Do I always do it the same way or do I vary it according to circumstances? If so, what circumstances?
- Have I tried to do it in a different way, and if so what happened?
- Have I omitted to do it for any reason and if so what were the consequences?
- Do I do it the same way as my colleagues? With similar results or not?
- How do I know it works? Should I continue to spend time on it?
- Must I always do things in the same order to achieve the same result? If I change would there be a difference?
- If I spent less time on it or did it less frequently would the outcome be different?
- What are the indicators of its success?
- Can a successful outcome be directly attributed to a particular facet of care delivery or could it be something else?

Independent learning through contracts

Another strategy for learning independently is to develop and use a learning contract. Independent learning modules based on contract learning are becoming increasingly popular in curricula at pre- and post-registration level as they provide the structure in which experiential learning can take place. Overall, the use of learning contracts is expanding in Higher Education so providing many more students, particularly students of the professions, with experience of this mode of learning to promote independence. Independent learning through contracts is a strategy that can also be used to good effect after qualification to achieve identified learning goals within a given timeframe but in a fairly flexible way. Learning contracts can also provide the means for accrediting work-based learning (DfEE, 1998) where they provide evidence that learning outcomes have been achieved.

A learning contract is 'a written agreement, negotiated between a learner and a teacher or staff adviser, that a particular activity will be undertaken in order to achieve a specific learning goal' (Anderson *et al.*, 1996, p. 2). It should define learning outcomes to be achieved, the learning support required, the structure for assessing achievements and the time-scale for completion (DfEE, 1998). Learning contracts should encourage learners to take more responsibility for their learning and to use existing skills and experiences as a basis for new learning. A learning contract is a flexible medium for designing learning activity and incorporates a process plan that clearly identifies how learning will be achieved.

There are differences between a project and independent learning using a contract. In a project the task to be completed is the focus of attention and it is likely to be the organisation that benefits primarily from the goal-directed activity. In contrast, a learning contract exists for the benefit of the learner. The emphasis is on learning as an outcome and not necessarily on the completion of a task, although completion is a desirable outcome. A personal adviser or mentor may facilitate learning activity specified in the learning contract but will not manage the activity as a project manager might manage a project. The learner takes responsibility for ensuring his or her learning needs are met by working to the contract that has been agreed.

In a learning contract the following are specified:

- The learning objectives or goals to be achieved
- The support required and resources available
- Details of how learning goals or objectives will be addressed
- The timeframe within which goals or objectives should be achieved
- The nature of the evidence that will indicate when goals or objectives have been met
- The criteria to be used to assess the evidence
- The signatures of the parties involved in the contract

Anyone agreeing to work to a learning contract has to take an active role in the learning process. It is the learner who specifies the desired learning outcomes and the manner in which they will be achieved. This means that the learning strategies that are proposed for achieving the outcomes can be those that reflect the learner's preferred learning style. Learning contracts for a number of people might specify similar goals, but the process of achieving those goals may be different for each one as the learning contract is fine-tuned to the needs of each individual. The learning contract provides the structure, including timeframe, for completing a learning project, but allows the learner some flexibility in choosing the resources and mode of learning that best suits him or her in relation to what has to be achieved.

The following twelve steps summarise the process of working through a learning contract.

(1) *The learner's needs or gaps in knowledge or skills are clarified.* The process involves examining your existing strengths, knowledge and skills

and identifying your needs in relation to your future career activity. A mentor can help you with this task.

(2) *Learning outcomes are defined.* This involves specifying what you will achieve in terms of learning within the agreed timescale. The outcomes expected need to reflect the opportunities and/or resources available to you, particularly in relation to the time allotted for their completion.

(3) *Learning opportunities and resources needed to attain the outcomes are identified.* It is important to consider resources in the widest possible sense including people, literature, organisations, courses, technology and yourself as the learner.

(4) *The process by which learning is to occur is specified in a plan.* This will include the learning strategies to address each of your identified learning outcomes. The learning strategy may be different for each one. It is likely that the strategies you select will be those that match your learning style preference. However, if the learning contract specifies that you will expand your repertoire of learning strategies as part of the learning process then you might choose alternative modes of learning that will make different demands on you and encourage you to learn in different ways.

(5) *Responsibilities of the people involved are detailed.* The two main parties are yourself as the learner and your adviser, but a contract may also involve other people, for example a supervisor or a mentor. Although you will take prime responsibility for the elements of the learning contract, some learning activity may be dependent on initial activity by other people.

(6) *The timeframe for completion is determined.* This may be dictated by some external factors. However, if you set your own timeframe, it should reflect the extent of work to be completed and depth of learning that is expected. The timeframe agreed therefore needs to be realistic. It is easy to underestimate the time involved in planning and carrying out learning activities that relate to specified outcomes.

(7) *The criteria against which the achievement of goals is to be assessed are recorded.* The criteria will act as a checklist for the evidence needed to ensure that the terms of your learning contract are fulfilled.

(8) *The learning contract is signed by both, or all parties concerned.* This shows a commitment to the contractual activity.

(9) *The learning activities are undertaken.* As the learning activities are undertaken, new themes or interests can emerge. If these are allowed to interfere with your original plan then the timeframe for completing the activity might be affected. This is not to say, however, that you cannot diversify, or that steering away from the original plan to a new way of looking at the issues is inappropriate. Learning should not be constrained

unnecessarily. Your plans can be revisited and revised, and the learning contract should be dynamic and modified in the light of change. However, this should only be done with careful consideration of the consequences.

(10) *The contract is revisited and revised as necessary as the plans progress.* There could be all sorts of reasons why this might be necessary but the learning contract should not be so rigid as to prohibit a change where change is clearly indicated.

(11) *Outcomes are evaluated against the recorded criteria.* This part of the learning process involves reviewing all the evidence to see the extent to which your learning outcomes have been achieved. It is always worth asking questions about what facilitated their achievement or what inhibited the work if desired outcomes were not achieved, or not achieved as intended. This adds an extra dimension to the learning process.

(12) *Future needs may indicate a renegotiation of the contract.* As the learning progresses it would not be unusual for needs or goals to change. The learning contract is a dynamic mechanism that can be subject to modification. If you undertake learning by contract, both you and your learning adviser should agree the specification of the contract and to any changes to the contract that arise out of a redefinition of goals.

The depth and breadth of learning that might be expected would be predefined if contributing to an academic programme, such as one leading to a professional qualification or postgraduate degree. However, the depth or breadth of learning that comes from activity specified in a learning contract that is used purely for professional development may not be as stringently defined.

One thing to be aware of is that learning contracts, by their nature, require learners to organise their own time and effort. This can be daunting if an individual is not used to self-directed learning. It is also easy to underestimate the time that tasks will take to complete, especially if they are dependent on input from other people. Timescales can be challenged. The support from an advisor is crucial to the success of learning from this type of experience.

Although largely used for learning in academic contexts, a contract to guide work and achieve learning outcomes can be used as an effective means of staff development in the work place. Where it is necessary for an individual to achieve work-related goals it would be possible to put a learning contract into operation in such a way that it directly relates to a specific outcome for the organisation but focuses on the learning process for the individual. The project may emerge as a result of a performance review or an appraisal of work. The contract can be negotiated with a line manager and/or an adviser and each will sign it with the individual learner. Equally, an individual might suggest to the line manager a topic for exploration that might be carried out using a learning contract. Rather than let the activity drift and have no clear timeframe, a formalised learning contract could provide the structure necessary to guide the learning to a successful conclusion. The learning that has taken place can readily be demonstrated against the criteria originally set and should be seen as a process of continuing professional development. A proforma for a learning contract is provided in Fig. 9.1.

Placements, attachments and secondments

Fieldwork education and clinical placements are experienced by all students of the health care professions. Although originally based on the apprenticeship model where students were expected to observe and practise 'in the mode of' the supervisor, much has changed. Learning outcomes for the period of practice are now more clearly defined. The active participation of the learner in the placement is seen as crucial to the learning process. Through these clinical experiences learners are expected to gain the conceptual understanding of practice with service users. The experiences of practice are normally explored by the learner with a competent supervisor through reflective dialogue in order to promote learning. The development of clinical reasoning and professional skills is expected to result. This model used for learning about practice and for participating in practice can, however, be useful post-qualification to develop professional skills to a deeper level of understanding or to broaden perspectives on practice.

Attachments or secondments also provide opportunities to experience practice in different areas of employment. For any of these experiences to be beneficial in terms of learning, the placement, attachment or secondment must be set up as a learning experience with defined learning outcomes to be achieved. A mentor or supervisor should be identified who will engage the participant in reflective discussion about experiences to help to determine the learning that has taken place. The learning relationship should help participants to gain fresh insights into practice and define future learning needs. Learning should be recorded and evaluated against the previously defined outcomes. The records of learning provide the evidence of continuing professional development for a portfolio.

Jobswaps

Jobswaps can be arranged to support the learning and professional development of two people simultaneously. They should be undertaken within a clearly defined framework. Both secondments and jobswaps may mean that the individuals concerned work temporarily for different employers so continuity of conditions of service have to be negotiated and agreed. There are many advantages to swapping jobs. It is possible to gain insights into a different area of practice for a defined period of time. It particularly benefits those who work for different organisations but whose work is carried out in partnership for the benefit of service users. It can facilitate a real understanding of another perspective of the job, especially the organisational arrangements that impinge on

Learning outcomes to be achieved with dates for their achievement	Learning strategies to be used	Support mechanisms to be used (named people and other resources)	Measures of performance (evidence on which performance will be judged)

Signed . . . .   Date . . . .

(Learner)

. . . .
(Mentor or supervisor)

Fig. 9.1 Proforma for a learning contract.

the work. It is a way, for example, in which university lecturers and practitioners can develop knowledge of each other's role and develop or refresh skills that will be assets when they return to their original employment. Learning from the new situations should ideally be recorded in a diary for future reference and to show evidence of professional development.

Case studies

One of the exploratory activities often carried out during a placement or secondment is a case study. Case studies can form projects associated with clinical work or management processes. They are most likely to relate to new situations or problems experienced by the learner that have not previously been explored.

Extended case studies based on new material can provide a framework for organising and presenting evidence of learning. It is possible to compile a portfolio based largely on case studies in order to demonstrate continuing professional development. Case studies can also be carried out methodically and analytically to gain a deeper personal appreciation of the issues or they can be carried out with the rigour of a research project as Yin (1994) explained.

Case study research has particular features and a text such as Yin (1994) should be consulted in this respect. Clinical or organisational case studies, as project work, can still yield new learning.

An organisational case study could examine a service or agency that is different from the one in which a practitioner normally works, or one that has special features that offer opportunities for learning. The organisational case study could explore:

- The nature of the organisation, profile of its users and relationships between them.
- The mission, aims and goals of the organisation and the way in which they are reflected in organisational activity.
- The organisational structure and manner in which work is allocated through the system.
- Any special features of the organisation which demonstrate innovation.
- The effectiveness of the organisation in meeting its aims and goals.

A critical review of these features of an organisation, a service, or an aspect of service provision could provide real insights into different arrangements for care delivery.

A clinical case study can show direct involvement with service users for the purpose of demonstrating continuing professional development. It can explore the way in which users' needs are addressed, the reasoning processes that go into decision-making about their care management and an evaluation of the effectiveness of the chosen intervention. Compiling and presenting information about different cases is particularly useful to demonstrate maintenance of professional competence for continuing state registration as the knowledge associated with it is directly related to practice. A critical review of a case will not just show how the case was managed but will provide a critical commentary as a reflective evaluation of the case management process. Case studies can therefore be presented at two different levels, first as the study itself, and second as a case study with a critical review of the case activity. Both would show evidence of learning.

Choosing a clinical case study

Case studies involving commonly seen conditions and problems experienced by service users may be subject to intervention strategies that are defined in a protocol or critical pathway. From time to time, however, an unusual case is presented that requires rather more thought or a different approach and makes particular demands in terms of research, consultation, professional reasoning and decision-making. These are the cases that are worthy of consideration for case study work. An extended case study could address all facets of the case and provide an evaluation of the material presented as a critical review. In documenting the case, care needs to be taken to maintain confidentiality of the service user. No reference should ever be made to personal details that might identify the user unless, of course, the user has given written permission for this to be recorded. A structure for presenting a case study could be as follows:

- *Essential details of the individual.* Age, gender, occupation.

- *The background to the case.* This includes how and why the individual came to be referred, an historical perspective on the case and the current situation, including social context, in which the person exists. The aim is to present concisely as complete a picture as possible of the person and his or her circumstances.

- *User's story.* Each health professional in contact with the user will provide a perspective on the case informed by his or her professional remit and approach to the case. It is therefore important to balance this input with a perspective gained from the service user about his or her own situation, past, present and potential future.

- *Identified needs.* Formal interview and assessment procedures are likely to be undertaken to obtain the necessary information for planning a programme of care. Once information has been gained from the service user it will be evaluated to determine problems and needs and the way in which those needs might be addressed. The case study can present a critique of the assessment process and its effectiveness in identifying problems and needs. The information selected as being pertinent to decision-making and the rationale for judgements made can be highlighted.

- *Key factors that make the case different.* In order to help identify the learning that emerges from dealing with a case, it is advisable to summarise the factors that make the case different from others. This helps to clarify thinking and the expected outcomes of intervention.

- *Plan and key responsibilities.* A summary of the plan of intervention and the individuals taking key responsibility for those plans can be identified but it is also important to evaluate the evidence for the plan, where necessary detailing why other options were rejected and the rationale for proceeding in a particular way.

- *Consultation/literature review.* Here it is worth noting any consultation processes that have occurred, including consulting the literature or with people. In a particularly unusual case it might be necessary to seek information about, for example, the condition and its prognosis, known methods of managing someone with the condition and evidence of effectiveness of known intervention strategies. New material learned can be summarised as key learning points.

- *Programme implementation.* The strategy for implementing a particular programme of intervention needs to be explained and if changes occur to the planned programme the reasoning behind the decisions needs to be made explicit. The outcomes of intervention should be stated with an evaluation of whether the outcomes were as intended, or not, and any observations about why there was a variation.

- *Summary of learning.* The whole purpose of the case study is to demonstrate that the experiences that you have had with service users have produced new knowledge, insight and/or skills that you can draw on to good effect in the future. Perhaps you have learned to use a new piece of equipment or applied its use in a new way. It may mean 'learning by mistakes' or learning more about yourself and the way in which you make decisions. It may mean using existing knowledge and skills in new ways. Whatever learning experiences you have had, it is essential that they are captured and made explicit for reference purposes.

- *Possible application of new learning.* By the same process, and thinking about the future, it is worth noting how the new learning might be applied in other circumstances. Was a piece of information more crucial than you originally thought? Did something that you did work well or not as well as you thought, and is this going to affect your approach in similar circumstances in the future?

- *Future plans and learning needs.* Given that new learning has arisen from the case study, are there any longer term implications, for example, the need to return to study a particular issue arising from the case, the need to explore some aspect of the work in more depth, or the need to develop particular skills further? Identifying learning needs can be part of a longer term process of planning continuing professional development and undertaking it in a meaningful way.

One of the key features of writing case studies is that new insights can emerge just through the process of writing down the details in a descriptive, yet analytical and evaluative way. The thinking processes involved often prompt new lines of enquiry about the process from which new learning arises. Comparing cases and making observations about similarities and differences can also be useful.

Gaining formal recognition for prior learning experience

Gaining formal recognition for prior learning normally means seeking credit for learning that has already taken place often in situations other than the academic environment. Credit provides a means of quantifying learning achieved at a given level and verified through valid and reliable assessment. It is awarded to learners who have demonstrated that they have attained specific learning outcomes (DfEE, 1998, p. 30).

The concept of accredited prior learning recognises that learning can take place in contexts other than a formal academic setting. The learning outcomes that have derived from previously completed work (for example, projects completed in the workplace) are assessed against the learning outcomes specified in a named, formal educational programme. The prior learning has to reflect the same competency development that the named education programme would develop. If the prior learning can be matched to the programme requirements then it can be accredited. Once accredited, the prior learning can then be counted as the learning that would otherwise have been achieved through participating directly in the programme, and can contribute to the academic award.

When submitting work for accreditation of prior learning you should understand that it is your learning that is being assessed and accredited. It is therefore no good submitting a curriculum vitae or a list of attendances at study days and conferences. These do not constitute evidence of learning. Learning outcomes and competence achieved through different learning experiences must be evidenced. It may be that learning from a number of different activities may comprise the evidence of learning for only one of the outcomes specified in the academic programme.

Prior learning will only be accepted as a substitute for an element of an educational programme if the learning is current, relevant and assessed to be at the appropriate academic level for the academic award to which it is to contribute. Changes in practice happen so quickly that learning can become out of date and superseded by new concepts, so it is essential that prior learning offered for accreditation is current. Learning that is out of date is unlikely to count. The relevance of the prior learning to the academic programme will also be considered. It may only be counted if it equates to learning that would have been achieved in the academic programme.

The academic level of a course lays down what is expected of students academically and intellectually in relation to what they should achieve by the end of the programme. Any prior learning to be taken into consideration would need to be assessed against these expectations and verified as being at the equivalent academic level to the programme for which it is being substituted. Experiential learning is judged according to its relevance, academic level and how current it is by university staff.

Universities are becoming more flexible in their approach to accreditation and are thus offering students more ways of attaining an academic award. This approach recognises that valuable, valid learning can happen anywhere and that individuals should not shy away from learning opportunities that are non-traditional or those that are not organised through a formal academic institution. All can result in quality learning.

References

Alsop, A. (1997) Evidence-based practice and continuing professional development. *British Journal of Occupational Therapy* **60**, 503–8.

Anderson, G., Boud, D. & Sampson, J. (1996) *Learning Contracts – A Practical Guide.* Kogan Page, London.

Bailey, D. (1991) *Research for the Health Professional – A Practical Guide.* F.A. Davis & Co., Philadelphia.

Barnett, R. (1994) *The Limits of Competence.* The Society for Research into Higher Education and Open University Press, Buckingham.

Barnett, R. (1997) *Higher Education: A Critical Business.* The Society for Research into Higher Education and Open University Press, Buckingham.

Chartered Society of Physiotherapy Research Development Group (1996) Physiotherapy research and continuing professional development. *Physiotherapy* **82**, 504–6.

DfEE (1998) *A Common Framework for Learning.* Department for Education and Employment, London.

Dowie, J. (1994) The research-practice gap and the role of decision analysis in closing it. Paper presented at the European Society for Medical Decision-making, Lille, October 1994.

Drummond, A. (1996) *Research Methods for Therapists.* Chapman & Hall, London.

Eakin, P. (1997) The Casson Memorial Lecture 1997. Shifting the balance – evidence-based practice. *British Journal of Occupational Therapy* **60**, 290–4.

Edwards, A. & Talbot, R. (1994) *The Hard-pressed Researcher – A Research Handbook for the Caring Professions.* Longman, London.

Ferrier, B., Marrin, M. & Seidman, J. (1988) Student autonomy in learning medicine: some participants experiences. In *Developing Student Autonomy in Learning*, 2nd edn (D. Boud, ed.). Kogan Page, London.

Gray, J.A.M. (1997) *Evidence-based Healthcare: How to Make Health Policy and Management Decisions.* Churchill Livingstone, Oxford.

Henry, J. (1989) Meaning and practice in experiential learning. In *Making Sense of Experiential Learning* (S. Warner Weil & I. McGill, eds). The Society for Research into Higher Education and Open University Press, Buckingham.

Hicks, N. (1997) Evidence-based health care. *Bandolier* **4**, 8.

Higgs, J. (1988) Planning learning experiences to promote autonomous learning. In *Developing Student Autonomy in Learning*, 2nd edn (D. Boud, ed.). Kogan Page, London.

Kitchen, S. (1997) Research, the therapist and the patient. *Journal of Interprofessional Care* **11**, 49–55.

Margerison, C. (1994) Action learning and excellence in management development. In *Managing Learning* (C. Mabey & P. Iles, eds). Routledge, London.

Margetson, D. (1994) Current educational reform and the significance of problem-based learning. *Studies in Higher Education* **19**, 5–19.

Mumford, A. (1994) Individual and organisational learning: the pursuit of change. In *Managing Learning* (C. Mabey & P. Iles, eds). Routledge, London.

Payton, O. (1994) *Research: The Validation of Clinical Practice*, 3rd edn. F.A. Davis & Co., Philadelphia.

Rosenberg, W. & Donald, A. (1995) Evidence-based medicine: an approach to clinical problem-solving. *British Medical Journal* **310**, 1122–26.

Taylor, I. (1997) *Developing Learning in Professional Education*. The Society for Research into Higher Education and Open University Press, Buckingham.

Taylor, M.C. (1999) *Evidence-based Practice for Occupational Therapists*. Blackwell Science, Oxford.

Yin, R.K. (1994) *Case Study Research*. Sage Publications, London.

Young, T. (1996) *How to be a Better Project Manager*. Kogan Page, London.

Chapter 10
Learning Skills and their Application

Developing skills for learning

Not only are learning strategies important, so are learning skills. Having the skills to learn effectively and the ability to translate experiences into learning enables you to add to your store of knowledge. Through new learning you can integrate new with existing knowledge and explore ways of applying new knowledge in different ways and in different contexts and situations. Knowing how to gain insights and identify the learning that has taken place through experience are key processes related to learning. The ability to ask questions effectively and to evaluate constructively work that you or other people have undertaken are also skills that can be developed to support the learning process. These skills underpin many activities through which you can work and learn. The process of reflection forms the basis of so much learning activity that it is addressed first.

Using reflection

Much of the theory related to adult learning stresses the value of using reflection to discover the meaning of new experiences and the learning that has been derived from them. New learning and continuing professional development depend on how skilfully you can reflect on your and others' practice, to gain new insights, see new relationships, make new discoveries and make explicit the new learning that occurs. The process of reflection involves a series of mental activities that help us to determine what has emerged during an experience and was learned from it. Reflection, according to Boud *et al.* (1993, p. 9), relates to 'those processes in which learners engage to recapture, notice and re-evaluate their experience, to work with the experience and turn it into learning'. Revisiting the experience in our mind, taking note of key features of the event, exploring for ourselves what happened and what the consequences were, and establishing how this adds to, or changes, what we already know, is the essence of reflection. Through reflection you will be in a position to use insights gathered from past experiences in future situations.

Palmer *et al.* (1994) explained reflection in a slightly different way although the process and outcome remained the same. They said that reflection on an action is the retrospective contemplation of practice undertaken in order to uncover the knowledge used in a particular situation, by analysing and interpreting the information recalled. This allows the reflective practitioner to speculate on how a situation might have been handled differently and what other knowledge would have been helpful. It allows future practice to be changed in the light of new knowledge and insights into practice. Improving practice in this way justifies the time taken to contemplate on what occurred. Processes that improve practice align with clinical governance concepts, so they are not outside practice but integral to it.

It may not always be possible to revisit an earlier encounter or to use new knowledge to change a situation. However, any new knowledge gained from experience will be stored for future reference as and when a similar situation arises. It is worth remembering that reflection is not just a useful process through which to gain insight into what did not go so well in a situation, it can also be useful to reflect on positive encounters and to explore the possible reasons for things going well. Only by reviewing situations will we gain some insight into the relative effectiveness of our actions in order to make sensible judgements in future professional practice.

Schön saw reflection in two domains, reflection *on* action and reflection *in* action. As noted above, practitioners who reflect *on* action are those who make a systematic review of events that have happened to establish whether, and how, practice was effective or whether different practice might have resulted in a better outcome. Practitioners who reflect *in* action are those who make reasoned decisions to modify their actions while they are actually working, based on changing circumstances at the time. For example, a practitioner who is working with a service user who suddenly deteriorates, or who reveals new information about himself pertinent to the intervention strategy, will not necessarily continue with a pre-defined plan of action but will reflect on the new information and will change a course of action to accommodate the new knowledge or change in circumstances.

Reflection has long been held as a skill that practitioners need to develop and use in their practice. Fish & Twinn (1997, p. 52) saw it as 'systematic, critical and creative thinking about action with the intention of understanding its roots and processes'. Through these processes it is possible to refine, improve or change future actions. Any change will result from reflecting that a course of action could or should be different. Brookfield (1986) commented that it was crucial for professionals to engage regularly in periods of reflection. Through reflection, by themselves or with others, practitioners can explore strategies for managing contextual problems and ambiguities in practice. In a wider sense practitioners should also reflect on the changing nature of practice in its political and economic context, or in relation to theoretical or technological advances. It is crucial to be able to recognise when practice is outdated or no longer effective. Steps can then be taken to update practice and to reduce reliance on ineffective techniques. Brookfield went so far as to warn us of the potential danger of 'client abuse' if professionals fail to keep abreast of developments. Reflection on practice in all its aspects is therefore not just good practice but essential for the well-being of all service users. Time spent on reviewing selected events or contextual circumstances will never be wasted. Any learning outcomes emerging from the activity, and the recommendations for modification to practice, could be presented in your CPD portfolio.

Asking questions

Asking the right questions in the right way underpins the process of learning, including the reflective activity through which learning occurs. Asking questions may be thought of as a fundamental activity yet asking questions effectively to elicit a response that makes sense is both an art and a skill to be learned. Questions have various functions. For example, they can help to:

- Gain feedback
- Explore phenomena
- Make sense of situations
- Elicit explanations, clarification or opinions
- Gain new insights
- Develop interest in a topic
- Review or confirm existing knowledge
- Expand thinking
- Develop reasoning skills
- Find alternative solutions

As an active learner you can take responsibility for participating in the learning process through asking questions. Questioning can help you to review, check and confirm your knowledge and move forward with new levels of understanding. The different stages include, first, reviewing and clarifying existing knowledge and understanding, second, formulating relevant questions to address limitations in understanding, third, listening carefully to the response, and finally seeking confirmation of what has been understood by the reply. The process thus has a beginning (reviewing), a middle (seeking new knowledge) and an ending as new material is confirmed and integrated with existing knowledge.

The confidence and ability to ask questions underpins the processes of reflection, evaluation and learning. You can ask questions of yourself or of other people. In personal reflection you ask questions of yourself. In dialogue you engage other people and use the discussion as an aid to learning. Asking questions can be spontaneous or planned and structured. Spontaneous discussion after an event can be very rewarding. It helps to clarify intent, develop interest and move understanding to a deeper level. Asking questions as part of the process of supervision, however, needs to be planned carefully. Preparing questions in advance not only saves time but also helps you to establish the real issues that need to be explored and the relevant questions that you are going to ask that will be of maximum benefit. Setting the scene by reviewing your current understanding of the situation is good practice and helps you to take responsibility for and control of the session. Asking the right questions can help you to attain a new level of understanding on which to move forward.

Being critical

Barnett (1997, p. 97) asserted that the professional world is a multiple world full of alternative possibilities of strategy, action and communication. But in order to perceive alternatives the individual has to learn to be a critical thinker capable of generating new ideas. Becoming a 'critical being' involves developing critical thought, critical action and critical self-reflection. Through critical self-reflection people develop themselves, and through critical thinking they develop confidence in forming an opinion. The insight gained through critical practice and through thinking critically about practice allows individuals to develop more efficient strategies for managing the things they have to do. Critical awareness and the learning that derives from it can be developed in a number of ways, all of which can be classified as continuing professional development.

Reading critically

Blaxter *et al.* (1996) explained that a critical reader does not take what is written at face value but considers that there may be alternative views, positions or perspectives that could be explored. Critical reading therefore goes beyond mere description of what has been read. Reading critically enables individuals to develop opinions and personal responses to arguments. It might show where the author's perspective is lacking or where there appear to be gaps in the discussion. Drummond (1996) suggested that to debate and challenge the methods and findings of an article can be useful, however persuasive it may seem at first sight. There could always be another equally acceptable viewpoint or interpretation worthy of consideration and reading critically should lead to the development of alternative perspectives.

It is clear, then, that reading critically is different from just reading and it is going to involve time and a conscious effort to achieve its purpose. Drummond acknowledged that reading critically is a skill that has to be developed. In her book she elaborated on each component of a paper for review to show how to work through it methodically and how to question the relevance, currency and soundness of the material presented. Further reference should therefore be made to this text.

The ability to read critically has its merits. A summary of the key points emerging from the reading and a list of references with a related critique could be inserted into a portfolio. Remember to date it. In later reviews of the literature you might alter your opinion in the light of new findings and circumstances.

Forming journal clubs

Journal clubs are formed by a number of individuals who share an interest in a topic, speciality or profession. They are prepared to learn with each other through the process of reading and reviewing articles, using the technique of critical reading. The club meets regularly to review and discuss articles that members have previously selected and read. The group would agree either all to read the same article, or to read different articles on the same topic and then to explore the strengths and limitations and relevance to practice of what they have read. The ability to read critically and to draw out salient points for discussion is an asset. The skill can be developed through group membership and active participation at the meetings. The learning that arises through discussion and debate will add to the wealth of knowledge and understanding about practice, it can help provide the evidence base for practice, or may trigger research questions for further exploration.

Exploring and reviewing literature

According to Blaxter *et al.* (1996, p. 110) a literature review is 'a critical summary and assessment of the range of existing materials dealing with knowledge and understanding in a given field'. It provides insights into previous work and sets the context for new work. This type of activity can be useful to update knowledge about a given area of practice and can provide an opportunity to explore what other people are doing in the same field of work.

As a learning professional, you will regularly search out and be alert to new information about your practice and will seek to improve knowledge and areas of competence in order to continue to work effectively with service users. There will therefore be many instances during your professional career when you will need to consult books, articles and other literature about your work. This may include looking for information related to clinical work, care management or to new interventions or strategies for practice. It might also include searching literature on management theory and processes, theories of education and their application in practice or seeking material to underpin formal audit, inquiry or research. Consulting literature may do no more than improve understanding of, say, a medical diagnosis, or it may set the scene for a large, complex inquiry into the evidence base for a specific area of practice.

Drummond (1996) outlined reasons for searching literature as part of the research process. However, these could equally be the reasons for consulting literature to support practice. They are:

- To discover the extent of literature related to a field of interest
- To gain up-to-date knowledge that is relevant to the work that you do or want to do in the future
- To identify factors that could generate questions about practice

Steps to explore literature may include consulting a known reference text, visiting the library or undertaking a detailed literature search using various search methods and tools. If finding relevant literature is a problem then Drummond (1996) suggested that you might start by asking your colleagues or known experts, or by looking at references at the end of articles or other books you have found. Texts on research methods, such as those by Drummond (1996) or Blaxter *et al.* (1996), provide full details of how to carry out a literature search, so this will not be addressed here. It is very likely that every time you check the literature you will discover something new that enhances your knowledge and understanding of practice. You may even find yourself using this new-found knowledge in your work.

Searching for and reviewing the literature for examples of good practice and evidence of effectiveness can be a time-consuming activity. It is important that you recognise that these activities, which form part of your everyday work, are worthy of note in a portfolio as evidence of continuing professional development. A short entry in the portfolio should specify the reason for the inquiry into the literature, any definitions and explanations of new terms that you have found, and a summary of the way in which the new knowledge will be applied in practice.

Writing critically

Being critical in reading, in verbal discussion or in writing should not imply criticism but should be about making informed judgements after evaluating the evidence, and then making suggestions for alternative ways of viewing the situation. A critique should be considered and justified and should aim to improve understanding of the issues. The critique itself, after all, may later be the subject of critical interpretation and an evaluation by other people. Blaxter *et al.* (1996, p. 217) cite Taylor's (1989, p. 67) work on motives that govern academic writing. The different positions that can be adopted when writing critically can be summarised as:

- Agreeing with, acceding to, defending or confirming a point.
- Proposing a new point of view.
- Conceding that an existing point of view has merits but could be better qualified.
- Reformulating and providing a new version for a point of view.
- Dismissing a point on account of its irrelevance or inadequacy.
- Rejecting, rebutting or refuting an argument on reasoned grounds.
- Reconciling two positions that may seem at variance or retracting a previous position based on new evidence or argument.

Writing a critical review of material found through a literature search, for example, may help you to clarify the arguments and establish justification for existing practice, or to form reasoned proposals for developing new practice.

Writing book reviews for publication

Another way of developing skills and enhancing and consolidating knowledge is to undertake a book review. This involves reading critically, forming an opinion about the book's relative merits and preparing a short critique that makes judgements about the book's relevance to practice and its potential use by practitioners. The review is intended to inform readers about the content and quality of the book and whether it might serve as an effective resource. Methven (1988), in a very readable article on book reviews as an educational tool, claimed that reviewing books can be a worthwhile and rewarding activity and can provide a mechanism for continuing education and for keeping up-to-date. Cormack (1994) suggested that writing a book review can be an individual's first publishing experience. Success in writing for publication may give you confidence to write editorials or longer articles that require research to be carried out. Publication demands the ability to organise material, to make constructive observations, to formulate cohesive arguments and manage a discussion in a cohesive way. Writing books demands similar skills and the ability to work with large quantities of material in an organised way. It also requires tenacity to complete the task! All publication is likely to count as CPD activity.

Reviewing critical incidents

Tripp (1993, p. 24) suggested that the term 'critical incident' has its foundation in history where it refers to some event or situation that marks a significant turning point or change in the life of a person, in an institution (such as a political party) or in some social phenomenon. Incidents that are so critical in health care are rare. Nevertheless, some incidents do become 'turning points' or are sufficiently memorable to have made some kind of emotional impact (Lillyman & Evans, 1996) to warrant exploration. Changes in practice may be prompted as a result of new insights gained from the experience. However, insights only come from a careful analysis of what happened, and of cause and effect. Careful and thorough analysis of an incident may reveal the factors that lead to a particularly successful outcome. Equally, an analysis may reveal aspects that lead to unwanted results. Whatever the case, the new insights will inform future decision-making and practice.

The critical incident technique was described earlier by Flanagan (1954). He noted that an exploration of the factors that lead up to an incident, and of the consequences of actions taken, can reveal the characteristics of practice that should be encouraged to achieve a desired outcome, and those that should be discouraged to avoid failure. Describing and analysing critical incidents, or those events or clinical cases that have been particularly problematic, can lead to new understandings of practice. When an incident is analysed it can become invested with new meaning and result in some transformation of both understanding and practice (Tripp, 1993). Improved understanding should help practitioners to develop the 'best practice' to which all professionals should aspire.

The process of learning about best practice is likely to involve an audit of practice itself. Critical incidents or cases may provide the trigger for case audit. Cases that have been particularly expensive to manage or that have been managed in particularly difficult circumstances might also be useful to scrutinise to see what can be learned from them. Equally those with a particularly successful outcome in relation to the resources used can be explored to gain an understanding of efficiency and effectiveness measures.

The first step is to document a concrete description of the critical incident in some detail. A summary should then be made of the events leading up to the incident. The consequences of any actions taken should be noted. Assessing the implications of actions will lead to a greater understanding of what happened and can provide evidence of learning. Detail, according to Tripp (1993), is important. Detail can be developed in two ways – either through *focus* or through *enlargement*. Focus involves clarifying the whole picture by increasing the definition of the existing details, whilst enlargement concerns changing the size of the things in the picture so more of the picture is seen in less detail or less of the picture in more detail. Whichever option is taken, incidents, or particular aspects of an incident, have to be described in sufficient detail for them to be analysed. New insights emerge from careful analysis of the event.

Analysis involves breaking a complex structure into its simpler constituent parts in order to better understand its nature and composition (Tripp, 1993, p. 26). Analysis provides an assessment of the event – of what happened, what made it happen, what it did, what it felt like and meant, and why it occurred. Interpretations reflect what is learned from the analysis. The aim of analysing critical incidents and learning from them is to discover how professional judgement can be improved.

Critical incidents can be explored by an individual, a multi-disciplinary team or a uniprofessional group. The intention is to learn, not to apportion blame, so it is important for this to be made clear at the outset to alleviate anxiety among interested participants. Using critical incidents for learning, with a view to improving practice, can only be beneficial. A personal record of the learning that transpires from the analysis can contribute to a portfolio.

Clinical audit

Clinical audit has been described as a clinically-led initiative that seeks to improve the quality and outcome of patient care through structured peer review whereby clinicians examine their practices and results against agreed explicit standards and modify their practice where indicated. (NHS Executive, 1996). Barnett & Kemp (1994, p. 12) suggested that the term is used to describe not only activities such as checking standards or outcomes, but more widely to mean 'the gathering of information by asking questions, checking records and observing clinical practice, the environment or the use of resources'. So clinical audit could be said to be an activity commonly carried out with a view to ascertaining and improving the quality of the service offered.

Audit serves as a system of quality control to ensure that effective measures are being taken to improve standards of care. Audit therefore aligns very much with the clinical governance agenda. The term audit, however, can conjure up ideas that the activity, taken to its natural conclusion, is a way of establishing accountability for wrong-doing and there may be a sense of concern about its use. The term is derived from the Latin word *audire* meaning 'to hear'. So, far from being a negative activity, audit is a process through which people 'hear about' what is going on in the clinical situation. It is thus a process of learning from which everyone can benefit. According to Barnett & Kemp, clinical audit is 'a co-operative, multi-professional assessment of the efficacy, social acceptability and economic efficiency of the care and treatment of patients with a specified disease, disorder or disability'. It involves all professionals pooling their evaluations of the care process and determining lessons to be learned for the future. The recording of audit activity, as a learning activity, may have a place in a portfolio.

Preparing critical pathways

Critical pathways are an attempt to define the route and procedures that should be followed in the care management of service users who have a particular diagnosis or clinical need. A clinical care pathway has been defined as a description of key events in the process of care which should be accomplished to achieve maximum quality at minimal costs (Spath, 1994). The argument in favour of critical pathways has always been to make the best use of resources and to control organisational costs, whilst ensuring the best outcomes for service users. Preparing critical pathways is not an easy task, however. It involves:

- Selecting a diagnosis or commonly used procedure
- Defining current practice for those contributing to care management
- Examining variations in current practice within the organisation and in other organisations to determine best practice
- Identifying how things could be done more efficiently and effectively
- Specifying the processes involved and outcomes to be expected
- Implementing the pathway on a trial basis
- Recording data about the use of the pathway, particularly the variations and outcomes
- Analysing data to inform the evaluation process
- Modifying the pathway to reflect changes in practice

Anyone involved in researching common and best practice and describing practice as a critical pathway will have learned a good deal from their efforts in terms of both knowledge and skills. This learning too can be detailed in a portfolio.

The critical review

Details of the way in which case studies might be used for CPD were presented in the last chapter. A critical review of a case and its management will add a different dimension to the learning process and the evidence of learning for the portfolio. It should demonstrate learning in both a wider sense and to a deeper level of understanding. A critical review could be presented in one of two ways. A summary can be provided at the end of the case material that presents a critical review of the whole process of case management, highlighting the lessons learned. Alternatively the case study, in its various stages, can be presented on one side of a page with a critical review of each stage presented on the opposite page. Obviously, presenting a critical review of a case will place more demands on you but the level and quality of learning to result from the reflective, critical process may be significant.

Learning outcomes

The success of continuing professional development and the various learning strategies that it involves should be measured and recorded in terms of learning outcomes. These are the achievements from all the effort that is put into learning. Learning outcomes are the results of past learning activity or experiences but can also be the goals of future learning activity. A learning outcome has been described as an explicit statement of achievement about what a person knows or can do as a result of a piece of formal or informal learning (McNair, 1996), that is, as a consequence of a programme of study, work or other prior experience (Fenwick *et al.*, 1992). It is likely to be something that an individual can now do that he or she could not do before the experience. Alternatively, it might show a qualitative difference in the way in which something is done that was not possible before.

Learning outcomes can be either prospective or retrospective:

- they can be pre-set for a programme of learning; or
- they can emerge naturally from unplanned or incidental learning experiences

For example, learning outcomes might be prescribed in advance if planning a workshop or a course of study, or when formulating a learning contract. The established learning outcomes structure the learning process and keep activity focused on what is to be learned. Although key learning outcomes may be specified in advance, these may not be the only outcomes that arise from an event. Other, more significant, learning may emerge incidentally and this can be translated into learning outcomes and recorded as such.

Learning outcomes arising out of previous experiences would not normally have been pre-defined as goals. These learning outcomes are statements that describe learning emerging from incidental or unplanned experiences but which nevertheless serve as learning experiences. Whether from pre-defined or incidental learning, knowing what has emerged as new learning can help individuals to determine gaps that remain in their knowledge and skills, and thus devise future learning plans.(Fenwick *et al.*, 1992).

Writing up learning outcomes

Learning outcomes are written in a particular form of language (McNair, 1996). They provide clear statements against which evidence produced by an individual can be matched in order to determine whether or not he or she has achieved the outcomes specified. Writing about learning outcomes can seem like a daunting task until you realise that it need only be about sentence completion. Examples of how to write learning outcomes are presented here for reference.

Pre-set learning outcomes that form part of a curriculum are likely to be preceded by:

> *By the end of the course, students will be able to ...*
> for example,
> *... collect, analyse and use data to plan a programme of care.*

Learning outcomes which form part of a learning contract might start with:

> *On completing this contract I shall be able to ...*
> for example,
> *... prepare a profile of users referred to the service for treatment.*

Learning outcomes arising from experiential learning might start with:

> *As a result of this experience I can now ...*
> for example,
> *... describe similarities and differences in the approaches to care management used by members of the team.*

Table 10.1 provides a list, by no means all-inclusive, of possible verbs that define actions for learning outcomes. The statements reflect competencies that can be assessed. They also provide the criteria for assessing prior experiential learning. You will note that a verb is used to state what is to be done. Writing learning outcomes for forthcoming or retrospective learning is fairly straightforward once the pattern for writing the outcomes is recognised.

Some other hints for writing learning outcomes:

- Be specific about the outcome that is to be, or has been, achieved
- Express the outcome in positive terms
- Consider the outcome to be the result of doing something
- Express the outcome in a way that can be assessed – to know whether it has been achieved
- Avoid terms that are difficult to assess e.g. *'understand'* or *'become familiar with'*
- Keep the statements clear and concise and avoid repetition
- Do not confuse process with outcome
- Check that learning outcomes that are to be achieved are indeed achievable

Table 10.1 Words used for writing learning outcomes.

act	formulate
address	fulfil
allocate	generate
analyse	identify
apply	initiate
appraise	instruct
argue	integrate
arrange	interpret
assess	interview
carry out	investigate
classify	justify
collate	list
comment on	make a judgement about
communicate	manage
compare and contrast	monitor
compile	negotiate
complete	organise
consolidate	outline
construct	participate in
contribute to	plan
create	practise
critique	prepare
debate	prescribe
define	present
demonstrate	produce
describe	provide
design	recognise
determine (e.g. strengths and limitations)	record
develop	reflect on (e.g. observations, experiences)
devise	relate
direct	report on
discriminate between	research
discuss	review
display	seek information on
distinguish between	select
draw on	show
draw together	solve problems
educate	specify
employ	state
enable	summarise
engage in	take account of
establish	take responsibility for
evaluate	teach
examine	trace
explain	use
explore	utilise
facilitate	write

Learning outcomes can relate to:

- The acquisition of information, knowledge or theory
- The application of knowledge or theory
- The development of intellectual skills such as analysis and reasoning
- The development of personal skills, attributes or attitudes
- The development of technical or practical skills

Learning outcomes are concerned only with the achievements of the learner (DfEE, 1998) and are thus differentiated from aims and objectives which address goals and tasks, respectively.

Learning aims and objectives

Learning aims and objectives are different from learning outcomes even though they all have a bearing on the end result of learning.

Aims of a project or programme of learning are general or global statements of intent or the overall goals to be achieved. One or two aims normally suffice for a project or learning experience.

Objectives are more numerous and provide more detail than aims. They specify the tasks to be done and give direction to the activity in order that the aims or goals can be achieved. For example, the objectives of a project might be to:

- Explore literature related to the topic
- Consult with identified experts in the field
- Examine critically known models of intervention
- Identify alternative strategies for addressing the problem

Outcomes, as indicated in the previous section, state what will have been achieved as a result of all the activity or tasks detailed in the objectives.

You should be aware, however, that other texts may give different definitions for aims, objectives and outcomes and lead to inconsistencies in application.

Evidence of learning

The assessment of continuing competence or the assessment of learning for accreditation purposes requires evidence of learning. Expressing learning in terms of outcomes from learning experiences can help the learner and the assessor to focus on appropriate material. The material provides the supporting evidence of learning and can be presented in many forms. The evidence must relate to the goals that were to be achieved. It is up to the learner to demonstrate the links between the identified goals and the evidence presented. Learning contracts or personal development plans offer ways of planning learning and of presenting evidence so that learning can be assessed against pre-defined criteria. Experiential learning, expressed in terms of learning outcomes (particularly where learning has to be identified for accreditation), will need supporting evidence to demonstrate that learning has taken place. Some of the types of evidence that might be considered are shown in Table 10.2 but an explanation of the evidence in relation to learning may still be required.

Table 10.2 Examples of evidence of learning or development.

abstracts	models
academic certificates or awards	papers prepared for presentation
articles	personal reflections
audit reports	photographs
bibliographies (annotated)	posters prepared for presentation
books	projects
book reviews	protocols or procedures
business plans	publications
case stories	published reviews of work undertaken
case studies	reference material
certificates of accredited learning	references
critical incident reviews	reflective diaries, journals or logs
critical reviews	reports
curricula of courses designed	research reports
diagrams (annotated)	reviews of development plans/learning
diaries	contracts
essays	standards documents
evaluations	systematic reviews
information leaflets	testimonials
learning logs	training manuals or resources
letters	videos
literature reviews	

Presenting the evidence

It is crucial that evidence of learning, learning outcomes and any assessment criteria are cross-referenced, particularly where a portfolio is submitted for assessment of prior learning. In this case it is advisable to create a portfolio specifically for the purpose of demonstrating that learning has taken place in relation to the given criteria. The relevant material can be pulled out of the main portfolio and assembled for a specific purpose. It is a good idea to put a table at the front of the portfolio that lists the criteria on which judgements are to be made, the learning outcomes that are relevant and offered for assessment, and any supporting evidence.

Learning strategies, learning skills and opportunities facilitate high quality learning. Knowing how to write learning outcomes allows this learning to be captured and recorded for filing in the portfolio.

References

Barnett, D. & Kemp, N. (1994) *The A-Z of Applied Quality for Clinical Managers in Hospital.* Chapman & Hall, London.

Barnett, R. (1997) *Higher Education: A Critical Business.* The Society for Research into Higher Education and Open University Press, Buckingham.

Blaxter, L., Hughes, C. & Tight, M. (1996) *How to Research.* Open University Press, Buckingham.

Boud, D., Cohen, R. & Walker, D. (eds) (1993) *Using Experience for Learning.* The Society for Research into Higher Education and Open University Press, Buckingham.

Brookfield, S. (1986) *Understanding and Facilitating Adult Learning.* Open University Press, Milton Keynes.

Cormack, S. (1994) *Writing for Nurses and Allied Professions.* Blackwell Science Publications, London.

DfEE (1998) *A Common Framework for Learning.* DfEE, London.

Drummond, A. (1996) *Research Methods for Therapists.* Chapman & Hall, London.

Fenwick, A., Assiter, A. & Nixon, N. (1992) *Profiling in Higher Education – Guidelines for the Development and Use of Profiling Schemes.* Council for National Academic Awards, London.

Fish, D. & Twinn, S. (1997) *Quality Clinical Supervision in the Health Care Professions: Principled Approaches to Practice.* Butterworth Heinemann, Oxford.

Flanagan, J.C. (1954) The critical incident technique. *Psychological Bulletin* **51**, 327–58.

Lilleyman, S. & Evans, B. (1996) *Designing a Personal Portfolio/Profile: A Workbook for Healthcare Professionals.* Quay Books, Dinton, Salisbury.

McNair, S. (1996) Learner autonomy in a changing world. In *Boundaries of Adult Learning* (R. Edwards, A. Hanson & P. Raggatt, eds). Routledge, London.

Methven, R.C. (1988) The book review: an educational tool. *Midwifery* **4**, 133–7.

NHS Executive (1996) *Clinical Audit in the NHS. Using Clinical Audit in the NHS: A Position Statement.* NHSE, Leeds.

Palmer, A., Burns, S. & Bulman, C. (1994) *Reflective Practice in Nursing – The Growth of the Professional Practitioner.* Blackwell Science, Oxford.

Spath, P. (ed.) (1994) Clinical tools for outcomes management. Cited in AOTA (1996) *Managed Care: An Occupational Therapy Sourcebook*, p. 28. The American Occupational Therapy Association, Inc. Bethesda.

Taylor, G. (1989) *The Student's Writing Guide for the Arts and Social Sciences.* Cited in L. Blaxter, C. Hughes & M. Tight (1996) *How to Research.* Open University Press, Buckingham.

Tripp, D. (1993) *Critical Incidents in Teaching.* Routledge, London.

Chapter 11
Gaining Qualifications

The qualification ladder

Students now qualifying to practise in one of the professions allied to medicine will earn an academic award from the institute of higher education that hosted their professional qualifying course. The academic level of the professional award will vary. For the majority of practitioners these days, the qualifying award will be a bachelor's degree, mostly with honours. A small minority will gain a postgraduate diploma and an even smaller number may be awarded a master's degree linked to their professional qualification. Those gaining postgraduate professional awards will already hold the academic qualification of a bachelor's degree.

In contrast, many practitioners who qualified to practise in their profession some years ago are more likely to hold a professional diploma awarded by their professional body. The professional diploma, although affording the licence to practise, is not normally recognised by universities as equating to a bachelor's degree even though it may have taken three years to complete, and is considered to be more akin to a higher education diploma. Understanding the academic level of your professional award helps to establish where you sit on the qualification ladder and how you may progress up the ladder.

An explanation of the qualification ladder is needed in order to understand the notion of continuing professional education (CPE) and the opportunities available within the higher education system for continuing professional development. Figure 11.1 shows the ladder and the sequential nature of the academic awards that are studied at either undergraduate or postgraduate level. The highest award to be gained through undergraduate studies is the bachelor's degree with honours. Those who have a bachelor's degree may be eligible to progress to postgraduate studies. Postgraduate studies, as you would expect, make more intellectual demands on students. The academic levels at undergraduate and postgraduate level are explained below.

Academic levels of study in higher education

The term 'level' is a 'generic guide to the relative demand, complexity, depth of study and degree of learner autonomy that characterises the learning expected, irrespective of the subject and context' (DfEE, 1998, p. 33). In higher education,

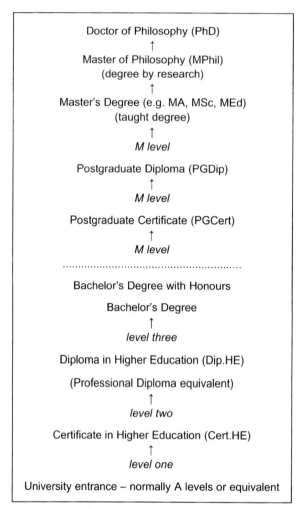

Fig.11.1 The qualification ladder.

levels are often, but not exclusively, categorised as *level one, two* or *three* for undergraduate studies and *level M* for postgraduate studies.

Undergraduate studies

All studies up to and including those for a bachelor's degree with honours will be pursued through a named university. These studies normally progress through the three different credit-rated academic levels, but the levels may or may not correlate with the academic year of study (for example, level one studies in year one, level two studies in year two). Programmes will vary in the way they are presented. Where a programme is delivered in modules, the credit rating and academic level of study should be indicated for each module.

Level one studies provide a foundation on which higher level studies can build. They normally contribute to a certificate in higher education. This is usually awarded after successful completion of the equivalent of one year of full time study of an undergraduate programme at this level.

Level two studies are at an intermediate level of difficulty. They build on level one studies and normally contribute to a diploma in higher education conferable after two years' successful full time study in an undergraduate programme. A professional diploma is normally deemed to be at this level.

Level three studies make conceptually higher demands of students, building on earlier levels of study. The final year of a full time undergraduate programme is normally at level three. A degree with or without honours can be awarded to students who are successful in their studies at this level.

The levels are fairly loosely defined. Each institute of higher education will have more detailed descriptors but these may vary between institutions. However, attempts are being made to establish a national framework for academic credit through a common framework for learning (DfEE, 1998), in an attempt to provide some consistency between universities. This should help students to transfer more readily from one institution to another and to have all current credits acknowledged by the new institution.

Each institute of higher education will specify its criteria for the achievement of either a bachelor's degree or a bachelor's degree with honours, the latter being a slightly higher academic award. Both will entail some level three studies although the honours degree will normally make quantifiably more demands of students. Normally, both the bachelor's degree and the bachelor's degree with honours can be awarded after three years' full time study. However, in some areas, for example in Scotland, a bachelor's degree with honours may only be awarded after the equivalent of four years of full time study.

'Top-up' degrees normally comprise the equivalent of one year full time study at level three to enable participants to bridge the gap between their professional diploma and the degree.

Modular programmes

A 'module' is a self-contained package of accredited study that defines the learning outcomes to be achieved, the indicative content, the teaching and learning strategies deployed, the reference materials required, and the mode of assessment used to verify that learning outcomes have been attained. Each module is given a credit value at an academic level stated by the institute of higher education that approved it. The level of academic credit is determined by the learning outcomes to be achieved, and the assessment criteria.

Individuals wishing to pursue academic study and who meet the entry criteria may often register for one single module or for groups of modules for CPD. Completion of a designated number of modules at specified levels can lead to a named academic award at undergraduate or postgraduate level. Increasingly flexible systems of learning allow for modules to be accessed at different institutes of higher education. Within a given regulatory framework, a cohesive selection of accredited modules can be accumulated from two or three institutions to be put towards an academic award from one of them (normally the institution through which at least half of the requisite modules have been studied).

Postgraduate studies

Taught degrees: Studies leading to a postgraduate award up to and including a master's degree are at master's level (often known as *M* level). Master's degrees may be taken full time or part time. Interim awards of a postgraduate certificate in higher education (PGCHE) and postgraduate diploma in higher education (PGDipHE) can normally be gained by those not wishing to pursue the full programme of study leading to the master's degree. If taken part time, the PGCHE would be awarded after approximately one year of successful study and the PGDipHE after two years of successful study. Studies up to PGDip level normally constitute the taught element of the master's degree. The full master's programme is completed through research and the preparation of a dissertation.

Research degrees: Postgraduate awards that involve study mainly through research include the Master of Philosophy (MPhil) and Doctor of Philosophy (PhD) degrees. These are undertaken either full or part time over a period of three to six years, working with one or more supervisors who help steer the work to a successful conclusion. The examination for both degrees involves preparation of a thesis which is a report of a significant piece of original research undertaken under supervision. A viva voce examination must also to be taken, based on the contents of the thesis.

Reasons for seeking higher qualifications

Understanding the levels of the different awards in higher education is important if you are to pursue a route to a higher qualification. However, there may be good reasons for gaining another award at the same academic level rather than aiming for a higher academic award than you already have. There can be different reasons for wanting to gain academic awards, for example:

- To develop intellectual skills and academic knowledge for personal gratification and reward.
- To undertake a focused, structured programme of learning with a view to upgrading professional knowledge and skills and maintaining competence to practise.
- To add to existing professional knowledge or skills, for example, by pursuing another recognised professional award such as a diploma in counselling and so provide wider scope for professional practice.
- To supplement the professional award with a recognised management qualification (for example the Diploma in Management Studies (DMS) or

Master of Business Administration (MBA) in order to progress a career in the field of management.

- To supplement the professional award with a recognised teaching qualification to enhance skills and to be able to facilitate learning in others.
- To pursue higher degree studies in a specialist area that might enhance practice and/or demonstrate higher level academic achievement. For instance, a master's degree is often required by anyone wishing to apply for a position as a university lecturer.
- To gain experience, under supervision, of carrying out research in order to be able confidently to seek evidence for best practice or to promote and support research within a service.
- To gain broader based knowledge and skills or a deeper understanding of practice and organisational issues to develop career opportunities or strengthen an application for career progression.

A higher education programme leading to an undergraduate or postgraduate award has been through a thorough process of vetting and approval before being implemented. It is audited annually through internal monitoring mechanisms and by external examiners in order to ensure the quality of teaching and academic rigour in course delivery. For this reason, universities will normally acknowledge the courses leading to recognised awards by other universities if students wish to transfer from one university programme to another. Employers can also be satisfied that university awards are of a known minimum standard (even though standards may vary) so that they can assess the merits of candidates with qualifications applying for employment. Employers can also assess the merits of supporting an employee through a university education programme for staff development. University education is thus generally recognised as meeting a known standard.

Higher education and continuing professional development

It should now be possible to see how gaining higher academic awards can be a route to continuing professional development. A structured programme, whether taught or pursued through research, can enable you to develop both personally and professionally. As a minimum outcome, a higher education programme should enable you to develop your knowledge base. However, the higher the academic level of the award, the more you are likely to develop and use intellectual skills, such as those used in reasoning, processing information, making judgements, developing arguments, skills in written communication and significant skills in criticism and evaluation. Anyone pursuing postgraduate studies can expect to develop intellectually so that they can apply new knowledge and skills in different areas of practice, not just in clinical areas but also in education, management and research. There is no doubt that undertaking postgraduate study helps an individual to develop confidence and both personal and professional skills. Those who undertake higher education are generally preparing themselves to be leaders in their profession.

Choosing a programme in higher education

It is probably true to say that never before has there been so much choice in courses leading to higher education awards. Most universities, and particularly those offering qualifying programmes for health professionals, will offer opportunities for higher academic study in areas related to professional practice. This is not to say that every health professional will want to continue to study at a higher academic level, nor that anyone wishing to study at a higher academic level will automatically choose to study a topic relating to practice. Choosing a course of study must be done as part of a carefully thought out career development plan that has been devised to reflect your future needs over a timeframe of at least three to five years.

In making a long-term plan for your future career moves, you would probably be well advised to seek help from or at least discuss your plans with a colleague or mentor who can act as a sounding board and help you to develop your ideas. Assuming that you wish to remain associated with your profession, or at least with health care delivery, the fields of employment that you might consider are likely to be in the areas of:

- Practice
- Research
- Management
- Education
- Consultancy or private practice

These areas are not mutually exclusive and it is possible to combine two or more of them. Knowing which areas are important to you and those in which you are least likely to practise will help you to focus your thoughts on higher education. You may well see advertised or hear of a course that sounds stimulating and is of interest to you and you may be tempted to apply. This is fine but you will be in a stronger position of knowing whether this is the right course for you if you have thought through your career development plan. You certainly need to think about the area in which you wish to be working in five years time so that you can pursue relevant (as well as interesting) studies. Higher education requires time, commitment and finance and so it is important to weigh up your options carefully.

Knowing how you learn best

Before making a choice in higher education it is worth thinking about the questions posed in Table 11.1. These questions may help you to form an opinion

Table 11.1 Learning preferences.

Mode of learning

- Do you prefer to learn with others or could you study on your own?
- Could you commit yourself to distance learning at home or would you prefer to have contact with others in the university system?
- Would you need regular, face-to-face contact with a tutor or could you organise your own learning and seek support as you need it?
- Do you need to work within a well-defined timeframe or do you prefer to learn at your own pace and at a time that suits you?
- Would you prefer to be taught on a course or to learn through your own research or investigation?
- Do you prefer to study full-time or part-time?
- Do you prefer day-time or evening study?
- Do you prefer to take examinations or to be assessed through ongoing coursework?
- What are your preferred learning styles and what learning strategies do you prefer? What modes of learning would you reject?
- What access do you have to academic programmes and will there be any practical problems (e.g. distance, transport, library access)?
- Will you be able to have study leave to attend a course in work hours or will you have to study in your own time?
- Would you prefer, or be prepared, to use technology to support your learning (e.g. web-based learning, tutorial support through e-mail)? Do you have appropriate access to resources?

Subject matter

- Are you seeking profession-specific, general or interprofessional education?
- Are you looking for course content related to a skill, discipline or client group?
- Are you looking for a course whose content is related to your career aspirations in clinical work, management, education, research or consultancy?

---

of the type of course that you might be looking for and about the courses that you would reject. It is important not just to think about geographical location and access, but also to think about how you like to learn and the importance to you of access to other people in your learning strategy. Some people are happy to be independent learners, others need the support and stimulation of a student group. Build up a profile of the type of programme that would suit you best. Analyse your preferences and needs carefully before you approach a university. The university prospectus should provide an outline of the course but do not be afraid to ask for clarification. The questions in Table 11.1 may help you to shape the questions you might ask.

Knowing your preferred learning style can also help you to make informed decisions about the type of education programme that might suit you. It is worth locating and completing one of the known learning styles questionnaires such as the one devised by Honey & Mumford (1992) to give an indication of how you learn best. No one style is better than another, it just helps to know how you learn best so you can be better placed to select modes of learning and academic programmes that allow you to use your strengths. People with particular traits show different preferences. Some people find that they have a mix of styles rather than one dominant style. This can be helpful as it allows greater flexibility in the selection process. Table 11.2 summarises some questions that may help you to discover your learning mode preferences.

Table 11.2 Learning styles.

Do you enjoy:
• Participating in something new?
• Tackling real-life problems?
• Participating in team games, role play, problem-solving groups?
• Generating new ideas, working beyond the constraints of rules?
• Learning from experience and opportunity?
• Having a high profile in situations – taking the lead, initiating discussions, giving presentations?
Activist-type
Do you prefer:
• To watch someone else before you have a go?
• To stand back, listen and watch events?
• To have time to think things over before making a decision?
• To be well prepared for making a contribution?
• To carry out thorough research?
• To assimilate information before drawing a conclusion?
Reflector-type
Do you like:
• Working with theories, models or concepts?
• To explore and probe the logic behind an idea?
• To explore relationships between ideas and situations?
• To be in situations where there is a clear purpose and direction?
• To be rational in an approach to something?
• To be challenged by complex situations?
Theorist-type
Do you like:
• To see the practical advantages of what you are doing?
• To see the links between the work to be addressed and the real work situation
• To have an action plan to work to?
• To try out ideas and work at improving with feedback?
• To use new ideas immediately in practice?
• To develop ideas for making a real contribution to an organisation's future success?
Pragmatist-type

Experience or qualifications?

University education provides a structure through which to learn and progress academically. It aims to meet the common needs of a significant student population. Successful completion of a pre-defined programme of study leads to a named academic award. This educational route is thus relatively straightforward and widely used.

Earlier in the book, however, the concept of experiential learning was discussed. Learning from experience is increasingly being accepted by academic institutions for accreditation towards an academic award. This means that a candidate may be required to compile a portfolio showing different experiences over time and how those experiences have contributed to learning. If the learning is assessed as relevant, it may be accredited. It is essential to remember, however, that it is *learning* that will be assessed and not the *experience*.

For many practitioners, learning from experience may be a preferred way of developing knowledge, skills and understanding of practice. It can be part of everyday practice and might be perceived to be less time consuming than a formal course of study. But learning this way tends to be less structured and it has to depend on the ability of the learner to establish a framework within which to focus learning in the context of practice, and then to produce the evidence of learning for ratification by the university.

For this to be successful, you have to set the agenda and the timeframe for learning. You have to make the judgement about what constitutes learning and how it is to be recorded. You have to organise the learning for yourself and keep yourself on track. This is very different from following a course of study that is all laid out for you – where someone else has pre-defined the learning outcomes that you are expected to achieve. An approved course defines the learning strategy through which learning should occur, the timeframe and the steps needed to achieve the outcomes, and recommends the texts that support the learning process. The assessment process of the course will enable you to demonstrate that you have achieved the learning outcomes to the level of understanding that is required. These elements are the fundamental components of a course of study. If you want to put together your own programme of learning then you have to follow similar steps. Some universities do allow you to follow independent routes of study where you set and agree the learning agenda with university staff. The university then provides the support and supervision needed as you tailor the programme to suit your own needs.

Will I be able to do it?

So often this is a question asked by those who lack confidence in their ability to study at a higher academic level. Anyone who has gained a professional qualification should, in theory, be able to cope with the demands of a postgraduate programme of study. The key is to want to do it. Some people find academic study challenging but enjoyable, others vow never to do anything beyond the qualifying examinations. So motivation is everything. The other aspect to consider is that in the professional qualifying programme there was a curriculum set by the professional body governing your practice. You had to follow the curriculum to gain the qualification and licence to practise. If you undertake postgraduate studies you can study a course that interests you and you can often follow options within the programme so that you are in far more control over what you learn and how you learn. This is the reason for asking yourself questions about your learning preferences, so you can find something that suits you. The choice is vast so there is bound to be something that you find interesting.

What if I only have a professional diploma?

Many people who have a professional diploma are satisfied with this award as it confers the licence to practise in their chosen profession. It was most likely awarded by the professional body as it confirmed competence in practice. A professional diploma can sometimes be more meaningful than an academic award and should certainly be something of which to be proud. But the questions often posed in the light of changes in initial professional qualifying education and in continuing professional development tend to stem from a feeling of 'being left behind' on the academic ladder and of inferiority when new practitioners qualify with degrees. There may also be concern that practitioners who hold diplomas may not be qualified to assess students who are working at undergraduate level. A question that is therefore often posed is:

Should I convert my diploma to a degree?

The answer to this question has to be one of personal choice. The key thing to remember is there is no *need* to convert from diploma to degree. Provided that you take steps to remain competent to practise then the question of the level of your award is academic. As a qualified practitioner, you will have been selected and trained to be a clinical supervisor or fieldwork educator because of your competence, expertise and experience in practice, and because of your ability to facilitate learning in the workplace. You will undoubtedly be expected to show that you understand and can apply theory to practice, that you base your practice on evidence of effectiveness wherever possible and that you can evaluate your practice and are committed to improving it as necessary. If you can carry out these activities you are certainly capable of studying for a higher academic award if you wish. You may, however, consider the second question:

As I only have a diploma, can I go straight on to postgraduate work or should I study for a first degree to begin with?

The answer is normally yes, you can go on directly to study at postgraduate level. However, there are still postgraduate programmes that expect applicants to have a good first degree with a classification of 2:1 or above. Equally, now that prior experiential learning can be accredited, universities are often prepared to consider alternative qualifications and other evidence of learning for access to a course. In this respect you will have to demonstrate that you can cope with the intellectual and academic demands of the higher degree. Evidence of learning and academic ability may need to be presented in portfolio form (see later in this chapter). Some universities may require you to submit an extended essay on a chosen topic in order to assess whether you can develop an academic argument. Other universities will accept the professional diploma in recognition of the rigour of the study involved. The onus will be on you to demonstrate that you have the ability to study at postgraduate level and that you are capable of passing the assessments.

Studying at undergraduate level first can seem a rather long-winded route to gaining the extra qualification as it can often take up to two years, part time, to gain the degree. However, if you lack confidence or have any doubts about your ability to succeed in academic work at a higher level, especially if you have not studied for some time, then there can be merit in returning to study at a slightly less demanding level. It can help you to develop confidence and additional study skills, especially in the use of library and learning resources, technology and the practice of searching for information. Developing research skills will also be useful as it is often assumed that the entry qualification of an honours degree ensures that the individual will have had practice in undertaking a small scale study. This is often not the case for those who have a professional diploma. The more that you gain practice in study skills the more adept you will be at tackling study assignments. This will put you in a better position to produce work at the higher academic level that postgraduate study will demand.

Learning alone or with others

Decisions about higher education and the type of course to pursue may be made on the basis of whether you prefer to work alone and in your own time at your own pace or whether you enjoy the stimulation of learning with others in a group at pre-arranged times. Most health professionals probably prefer to have contact with others for support and welcome the opportunity to engage in dialogue. Even the social support of a student group can be an attraction. Some individuals, however, prefer to study alone and at a time that best suits them in relation to other work and personal commitments. Some people may not have easy access to higher education so distance and open learning can be attractive in some instances. Teleconferencing and e-mail can provide the facility for dialogue at a distance.

If your preferred mode of learning involves working with other people then further decisions need to be made. For example, if the academic programme is profession-specific this will limit you to learning with members of your own profession. This may have benefits in allowing you to explore theory and practice to a deeper level of understanding as you will share a common language and similar knowledge from the start. However, exposure to other perspectives may be more beneficial and broaden academic thinking. Studying at postgraduate level with people from various professional backgrounds has different benefits.

Individuals can share knowledge and expertise and learn from each other. Interprofessional learning is well supported by the Government, as is team learning. There is no reason why an academic programme should not centre round the needs of interdisciplinary teams of service providers.

The mode of learning – alone or with others – is therefore a personal decision based on personal preferences, needs and interests. The decision has to be taken in an informed way after consideration of the various benefits and costs of the different approaches.

Flexibility

In planning a programme for yourself you can build in the flexibility that you need. There can be flexibility about how it is carried out, the choice of learning method, and when it is carried out. Knowing your preferred learning style may help you to decide which pathway to take. There are many ways of continuing to develop professionally by taking a keener interest in what goes on in practice. This book contains many examples of how that might take place and how everyday activities can be translated into learning. Provided that experiences are systematically reviewed through personal reflection, or in dialogue with other people, learning will become apparent. A portfolio can be built up from personal reflections and summaries of insightful conversations with other people about practice issues.

Making the effort to do this will require commitment, however, it is always easy to make excuses or to feel that other professional (or leisure!) activities should take priority. The flexibility of experiential learning can mean that learning becomes haphazard if you are not committed to the cause. Even more commitment is needed to record the experiences in terms of learning because this can be a difficult part of the learning process. Often, learning only becomes apparent when you actually try to write down what you have learned from the various experiences.

The way that you learn and ensure your continuing professional development is up to you. You may decide to make the effort and choose some experiential learning strategies, recording the learning outcomes that occur. Alternatively you may be someone who prefers to follow a structured programme of learning and to pursue academic qualifications that relate to professional activity. You may, of course, mix the modes of learning. All can be counted as continuing professional development.

Preparing a portfolio for accreditation of prior learning

If you are asked to present material to a university for assessment of prior learning then many of the principles of portfolio preparation detailed earlier in this book will apply. The purpose of presenting material in this way is for the course leader to establish whether there is sufficient evidence in your portfolio to give you academic credit for your prior learning. This can then be substituted for part of the course for which you are applying. This means that the prior learning that you have gained must equate to the learning that you would gain if you were to follow the programme of study. If you are awarded credit then you may be exempt from selected elements of the programme because it will be considered that you have already mastered them. In the process of examining your work there are certain features that will be assessed:

- The evidence of learning
- The relevance of the prior learning to the proposed course of study
- Whether the previous learning is out of date or is still current
- The academic level of the learning that emerges from the evidence

The prior experiential learning has to be at a level equal to the learning that would normally take place while doing the course. For example, if you want to pursue postgraduate study, then any accredited learning that is to count towards the award will need to be assessed at *M* level. If the learning has been assessed as only being at *level three* then it may not count towards a postgraduate award. The level at which it is assessed will reflect not just the new knowledge but also the evaluation and application of that knowledge in practice. Critical awareness of how that knowledge can be used will be needed for *M* level credit.

It is a very time-consuming business to put evidence together and demonstrate that this constitutes learning. The evidence has to be summarised and presented in some logical form and the learning outcomes extracted from the evidence. The evidence may come from certificated studies completed as part of another course. In this case, a transcript of learning outcomes should be available. On the other hand, learning that has arisen from project work or other similar, work-based experiences will need to be explained.

A good start is to ask whether there are guidelines for preparing evidence for assessment of your prior experiential learning. It is also necessary to have full details of the course for which you are applying for exemption. You will then see what you would have covered in the course and you can make some decisions about which material you select as evidence. It is important that your choice provides exactly the right evidence of learning for the particular component of the course for which you are applying for exemption. You must be selective. Not all material will be relevant – irrelevant material tends to show your inability to make judgements about what is relevant. Seek guidance by all means if you are unsure. You may find that you have not included a whole batch of material, but it does not matter as long as your selection is relevant.

Once you have the evidence that you wish to include in your portfolio you should present it in such a way that it is easy for others to access and assess. It may be that the material is insufficient in itself so you will need to summarise the evidence and the learning outcomes that emerged. As a rule of thumb, the finer and sleeker the portfolio, the more likely it is to show the evidence required. Some people think that the more that you put in the better and they produce enormous, weighty portfolios, but on scrutiny there is little evidence at all of their own work. The material may have been collected from a range of sources but it does not show evidence of *personal* learning. You have to work at it and make sure that you extract the relevant features that demonstrate learning specific to the criteria against which you will be assessed. Quality not quantity is the best way of summing up what is required.

It is also worth thinking about the assessor and the job that he or she will have in finding evidence in your portfolio and matching it to course requirements. You can help this process by providing a clear structure to the portfolio, an index, and by carefully laying out the material in sections. The relevance of the material should be indicated and pointers should be given to show how the material links with other sections. You should explain the nature of the evidence and how you feel that it demonstrates your learning in relation to the programme requirements.

As a summary, Hull and Redfern (1996) made some very pertinent points to remember:

- It is learning, not experience, that is being assessed.
- The learning that is being demonstrated needs to be sharply focused against the assessment criteria.
- The assessor needs to be convinced that the assessment criteria are met. It is essential not to put in everything known and available but only material carefully selected to match the assessment criteria.

There is no guarantee that the portfolio will be assessed as demonstrating that you have previously mastered the knowledge and skills that you claim. It may still be necessary, and may even be desirable, for you to complete the full scheduled programme.

The experience of higher education

Those who seek higher education most likely want to develop their skills and knowledge and to make a serious attempt to improve their academic qualifications. This is commendable, a situation where everyone can benefit – the health professional, the service and the service users.

Gaining a place on a higher education programme is relatively straightforward. Gaining financial support and study leave to take advantage of it is another matter. Funding for continuing professional education is limited for those working in health and social care and gaining agreement for study leave is difficult when all services are under pressure and resources are scarce. Personal commitment is essential and financial backing crucial if there is no access to other funds. Institutes of higher education are doing what they can to make programmes accessible. Part-time study and distance learning are available and evening study is possible, even if it is less attractive to students. Whatever the demands, however, the benefits to be gained from higher education are significant.

The experience of (re-)entering higher education can be daunting for some, but once there, the learning environment can be both stimulating and challenging. Higher education provides 'time out' of the work environment, away from its associated pressures to experience a level of personal and professional development that could never be achieved in-house. Meeting up with other people who also want to be challenged can enhance the academic experience. Having the opportunity to debate, question and hear other views can be exciting. The experience allows personal and professional growth as well as the development of intellectual skills. It promotes increased confidence, personal management skills and the ability to think creatively. It allows people to develop their true potential and to see how they might use their enhanced skills in the practice setting.

The experience of higher education is one to be savoured. Personal values and goals are likely to be redefined as there is a heightened awareness of personal capacity and capability. If anything, it can be frustrating to return to the same working environment unless there is some discussion about how newly developed skills might be used and put into practice. You will be a changed person from the experience, able and willing to move on to face new employment challenges.

Meeting the expectations of different people

The one thing to remember when undertaking a course of study, particularly a programme that leads to an academic award, is that you are doing it primarily for yourself. Funding for the course may come from another source, such as an employer, so it can easily, but mistakenly, be perceived that ownership of the project remains with the sponsor. This is not so. There may be an agreement or a commitment to a particular study topic that has benefits for the service, but the way it is approached and the slant that it takes will ultimately be for you to determine.

If a project is undertaken as part of an academic award then supervision for the project will come from an institute of higher education. The guidance given during the project will be aimed at achieving a successful result, that is, for you to gain the academic award. You will need to listen carefully to the advice of your academic tutor who will be in a good position to make recommendations to you about the range and level of activity that you undertake and the matters that you might address. This goes for the production of the final report as well. The primary report will go to the university to fulfil the requirements of the academic assessment. If that report is unsuitable for use in your service then you may have to modify it and produce a second report for a different readership. Tensions can easily arise where there is a lack of clarity about the locus of control of the project and, as the person in the middle of all the tensions, you need to be clear that you should retain control.

References

DfEE (1998) *A Common Framework for Learning.* Department for Education and Employment, London.

Honey, P. & Mumford, A. (1992) *The Manual of Learning Styles.* Peter Honey, Ardingly House, Maidenhead, Berks.

Hull, C. & Redfern, L. (1996) *Profiles and Portfolios: A Guide for Nurses and Midwives.* Macmillan, Basingstoke.

Chapter 12

Support for Learning and Continuing Professional Development

Finding support

While you have a responsibility as a professional for your own continuing professional development, it can be a distinct advantage to have access to people who are prepared to take an interest in what you are doing and to offer guidance and support. There are many kinds of potential support mechanisms, each offering something slightly different. It is worth considering which might be the most relevant to you and seeking out the support that is going to help you best with your learning. The following are sources of support that might assist with your continuing professional development. Each will be discussed in turn.

- Line manager
- Coach
- Mentor
- Peer
- Educator
- Clinical supervisor/fieldwork educator
- Professional body

Line management support

As an employee, you may think of your current post as a step or building block in an unfolding career. The job provides satisfaction and personal rewards but also acts as the basis for developing your professional skills and prepares you for new roles. One job thus acts as a stepping stone to another, a rung on the career ladder. In your capacity as an employee, a natural working relationship exists between you and your line manager. Hopefully your line manager is facilitative of your professional and career development within the service. For a service to be effective and delivered to the highest standard, staff competence, motivation and satisfaction are paramount. Maintaining standards means maintaining the competence of the workforce but it also helps if staff are contented and motivated to do the work that they are required to do.

Motivation and satisfaction tend to arise as a result of the support that employees gain from managers in their endeavours to develop competence and professional expertise. The support that you can expect from a line manager is important, but it is likely to be limited largely to what is essential for service provision. Your professional development will be targeted to ensure that you remain competent in your job and so that you can continue to contribute effectively to service delivery. One role, however, that of the coach, can be concerned with both line management and the facilitation of your learning so that your individual as well as organisational needs are addressed. In a different capacity, a mentor can offer support and guidance to individuals separate from line management and preferably at a distance from the workplace. Both these roles are explored in more detail shortly, but first it is necessary to consider performance review as a process of determining what needs to be achieved by the employee as a learner and a member of staff.

Performance review

A service concerned with quality and effectiveness is likely to have a system in place for a formal, periodic review of staff performance. An appraisal or individual performance review (IPR) system operates to guidelines produced by the human resources department of the service. It is a systematic way of identifying individuals' strengths and needs and for ensuring that staff competence and expertise are developed and used to the best advantage for service provision. By April 2000 the majority of health professional staff employed within the Health Service should have a personal development plan (PDP) (Department of Health, 1998).

As a member of staff you will be asked to participate in the performance review system, probably once a year, in order to:

- Review your recent performance and the extent to which your previously established goals have been fulfilled.
- Acknowledge good performance and evaluate its relevance to service delivery.
- Discuss any areas of concern or difficulties that you encountered in achieving the previous year's goals.
- Identify current trends in relation to the skills and competence you need to have to support service delivery.
- Negotiate and set new, service related, goals that you agree to work towards meeting within an agreed timeframe.
- Establish the plan of how goals are to be achieved.

More enlightened line managers may set the action plan in the context of your career development so that there are gains for both you and the service. Enabling you to develop the skills to move into new roles might support a wider staff retention strategy that enables all staff to work towards promotion or to take additional responsibilities within the same employing organisation.

The review process

Your line manager will normally conduct the review but you should take an equal and active part in the preparation and discussions, and in the formulation of the action plan which sets out your personal agenda for the forthcoming year.

Preparation normally involves revisiting development plans and goals set at the last performance review meeting to ascertain the extent to which these have been addressed and achieved. Sometimes a form has to be completed by both reviewer and reviewee. This should note achievements against goals and any significant changes in practice or in the context of practice that have affected, or are currently affecting, performance. Limitations in competence or possible gaps in ability need to be highlighted. Your performance should also be reviewed against your job description. The review may indicate that your job description needs changing to reflect more accurately your current role in the service.

Discussion should be a two-way, constructive exchange of information and ideas. Ideally, you, as the reviewee, should first offer an evaluation of your own performance over the period of review. This allows you to identify strengths and achievements and to explore significant factors that have facilitated your performance and a satisfactory outcome of goals. It is important to reflect on the positive aspects of your performance first and to have those confirmed by your line manager. These discussions tend to demonstrate that, despite any service changes and environmental factors that have influenced your activity, positive developments have taken place and are worthy of note.

Exploring elements of practice that have been less successful should be tackled next. An honest critique of your performance, first from you and then from your reviewer, should lead to an open discussion about any factors that have inhibited performance and resulted in a less satisfactory outcome than expected. Constructive comments about the situation are to be encouraged so that hopes and plans for the future can be identified. There may be valid reasons for the outcome, which should be noted. These may indicate that a shift of focus is needed in relation to your future goals.

Future plans and goals should be negotiated jointly. An action plan should set out the future direction that any developmental activity should take, and should reflect your service needs and organisational goals. The plan should also reflect the expectation that you must remain safe and competent to practise in your position of employment. There are potentially three areas that can be addressed in the action plan:

- Goals that enable you to maintain competence to practise
- Goals that support service needs and developments
- Goals that support your career development needs

The first two sets of goals will be of primary interest to the service and are likely to underpin the action plan. However, employers could also acknowledge your personal career interests and support these wherever possible as a commitment to the staff retention strategy of the service. The Government has advocated that career aspirations as well as service requirements, should be addressed, when continuing professional development is planned (Department of Health, 1999).

Formal notes of the performance review can be kept in the 'private' section of your portfolio for future reference. They should demonstrate that you have participated in the review process and have set goals for the next year. The goals established at the time of the performance review may only be service-related so you may wish to add your own personal career development goals to them. The plan may include activities that are intended to enhance your competence and performance in order to improve the effectiveness of service delivery. Plans associated with your performance review can thus lead to your continuing professional development and should attract the support needed from managers to carry them through.

Implementing your personal and professional development plan

Performance review systems can help you to reflect on your contribution to service provision and identify your learning needs in the light of your current and future responsibilities within the organisation. In the course of the performance review, your line manager may acknowledge your learning needs and formally note them in the development plan, along with a scheme for addressing them. However, managers may not always be in a position to facilitate your programme of development. If your manager agrees to coach you then this will be built into the plan. Otherwise you may be left to your own devices to implement the plan and monitor its effectiveness in meeting your goals. Learning mentors can be appropriate people to assist you under these circumstances.

Working to short-term personal and professional development goals that align with service plans can readily be achieved, but service needs and goals tend to be the drivers of staff development plans. For this reason you, as an employee, need to take time every so often to reflect, not only on your professional development but also on your personal plans and the overall direction of your future career. Your longer term goals for career development need to be identified and you should put a strategy in place for ensuring that your personal aims and goals can be achieved. This, again, is where a mentor might help you. Coaching and mentoring are two possible support mechanisms that can help you to achieve your goals.

Coaching and mentoring

In some texts the terms 'coach' and 'mentor' seem to be used interchangeably but Parsloe (1995) made it clear that there are two distinct roles. These are described here to distinguish between the different types of support that might be available to you, and what you might expect of them. Parsloe (1995) noted the origins of both words as a useful starting point. Coaching, he suggested, is derived from university slang for private tutoring or instruction in sport, whereas mentoring has its origins in advising and counselling. Coaching is therefore directly concerned with the immediate improvement of performance and development of skills, whereas mentoring is concerned with the longer term acquisition and application of skills in a developing career.

Both a mentor and a coach can facilitate your learning but the opportunities for, range and direction of learning might be different. Both can assist you with a vision of your future and help you to develop your skills to achieve your ambitions and goals. A coach, however, is likely to be your line manager or someone who has direct contact with you in the workplace so that the process of your skill development takes place within the context of service provision. A mentor, on the other hand, may be a friend within or outside the service who acts as a sounding board for you, rather than as a supervisor of your professional activity. A mentor in the workplace is always one step removed from direct line management responsibility (Parsloe, 1995). The one limitation of the coaching process is that it ceases when either of the employees leaves the service. Mentoring, however, is a more overarching process concerned less with detail and more with an overview of your development. The same person can remain your mentor however many times you change jobs which can provide continuity of support for you in your transition from one job to another. One distinction in particular was noted by Megginson & Pedlar (1992, p. 51) who commented, 'where coaching builds performance, mentoring is concerned with building a life's work'.

If your employers acknowledge your need for either a coach or a mentor and support you in your efforts to fulfil it, the organisation is demonstrating its commitment to the development of its staff.

Having coaching

Coaching is said to be a process in which 'a manager helps a member of staff to solve a problem, carry out a task or complete a task better, through discussion and guided activity' (Kalinauckas, 1995, p. 133). This involves exploring an opportunity or a problem together and enabling the learner to develop new knowledge, skills and competencies in working independently on it (Megginson & Pedlar, 1992, p. 50). The learner is expected to play the greater part in these activities, with support and assistance where necessary.

Coaching uses the process of modelling, exposing the learner to the way in which an expert thinks, reasons and makes decisions. Reflection on the process facilitates learning and the integration of new knowledge and skills into subsequent practice. The focus of coaching, according to Kalinauckas, is on practical improvement of performance and on the development of specific skills. He goes on to describe 'achievement coaching' as a continuous and participative process whereby the coach provides both the opportunity and encouragement for an individual to address his or her needs effectively in the context of personal and organisational objectives. This suggests that the process of coaching starts with the individual's agenda for learning, which is somehow dovetailed into the arrangements for meeting service objectives. The process of clinical supervision is similar to coaching in many respects, except that an assessment of performance is undertaken at the end of the clinical or fieldwork education programme.

Reference to relevant literature (Megginson & Pedlar, 1992; Parsloe, 1995) suggests that the coach might be expected to do the following:

- Help clarify learning goals and set targets
- Talk through the task
- Enthuse about the work
- Demonstrate competence
- Demonstrate the use of relevant technology
- Give good attention
- Recognise skilled behaviour
- Give feedback
- Help explore and use mistakes constructively
- Encourage self-monitoring
- Respond to doubts

Kalinauckas (1995) asserted that coaching is about bringing out the best in people through an exploration of their personal vision, values and beliefs and linking these to the vision, values and beliefs of the organisation. Everyone should gain from the process because the employee is working to achieve the same goals as the service so that users benefit yet coaching allows the employee to realise his or her potential in the process.

Working with a mentor

A mentor is someone dedicated to the personal and professional growth of another (Javernick, 1994), someone sought out for being able to develop a person's knowledge, skills and aspirations. A mentor is concerned with an individual's journey through his or her career. An experienced mentor can listen to, encourage, guide and support an individual in developing a career pathway according to personal expectations, interests and goals, and help the individual to determine the plans to pursue them. A mentor needs to have a store of ideas that can be drawn on to help an individual to devise and use strategies to meet personal goals. The mentor will have access to information and resources or knowledge of learning opportunities that can be tapped into for learning and development. He or she might also have a well-developed philosophy of life and an ability to operate on a spiritual dimension as well as at an intellectual and emotional level (Megginson & Pedlar, 1992).

A learning mentor has a very different relationship with an employee than a line manager. The mentor's relationship is facilitative but non-directive. It focuses on the employee's needs, rather than on the needs of the service or service user. Burdett (1994) saw it as a role that uses dialogue to facilitate problem-solving and learning. Using someone from outside the service can bring objectivity to discussions. He or she will have the capacity to look beyond the service for opportunities for learning and career development. It is thus a much broader role than that of a coach.

Daloz (1986) suggested that a good mentor is concerned with three particular objectives:

- Supporting you
- Challenging you in discussions
- Shaping the way you aim to achieve goals, and providing a vision to help you map out your future

Your career is a matter of personal choice. Self-monitoring and self-evaluation of your career progress are commendable activities and may lead to new insights about the future direction of your work. However, a career can be more effectively planned with the help of someone who has a real interest in you as a person and in your abilities and goals for the future. A mentor is someone who can be a sounding board for your ideas, who can assess your strengths, challenge your assumptions, work with you to explore your concerns and help you to develop effective strategies for career development. Clearly this has to be a person you trust and respect but it also has to be someone who will empower you to find the best route for your career. A mentor does not necessarily have to be someone from the same profession as you, more someone able and willing to work in a close relationship with you to facilitate your development and growth. The access that you have to your mentor and the relationship that you have with him or her will be crucial to the success of the mentoring activity.

If you should feel that having a mentor might assist you in your development, it is important for you to be able to ask someone who you respect to act in that capacity. You should select a mentor for yourself because the quality of the relationship is the crucial factor in the success of mentorship. Although your manager might have some ideas and suggest people who you might approach, there should be no compulsion for you to accept the manager's suggestion. You must be able to decide for yourself who is likely to facilitate your learning and development.

Whether as an informal or formal arrangement, being mentored offers an extremely valuable support mechanism for anyone seeking to develop themselves personally and professionally. The mentor should be a good listener and might be expected to:

- Help you to develop a vision of your future career
- Be a good listener

- Be a sounding board for your ideas
- Enable you to recognise your assets as well as gaps in your experience
- Facilitate the exploration and development of your ideas
- Enable you to determine a direction for future professional development
- Enable you to manage the process of CPD
- Aid your reflection on the process and progress of your CPD
- Help you make sense of situations
- Offer suggestions about opportunities or resources to support your development
- Offer suggestions about additions to your portfolio

In the mentorship relationship, it is essential for you to negotiate the parameters of the arrangement with your mentor, such as the following:

- How frequently you meet
- Where you meet (formally at work or informally over a coffee or a drink)
- The most acceptable arrangement for contacting your mentor (at home, at work, in or outside office hours)
- Whether weekends are included or excluded from the arrangements
- The permitted and excluded agenda items
- The confidential nature of the business
- The relationship between your mentor, your manager, and yourself

It should also be accepted that the mentoring role is not a counselling role. Whilst issues pertinent to your professional development and growth may be discussed, such as barriers to learning and to progress, these should be confined to those that are professionally relevant rather than include matters of a purely personal nature. Both you and your mentor need to respect the parameters of the role in order to maintain the quality of the relationship and the focus of support. The primary focus of mentorship can encompass all facets of personal and professional development, and this may include career development in its widest sense and not just related to current employment. The focus of support will thus differ from that which you have with your line manager, where the purpose is likely to be narrower and more focused on service delivery.

Peer group support

Support from colleagues at work, from those working in different services but in the same clinical field or from colleagues who are on the same course of study, can be extremely valuable. Colleagues serve as a point of reference for questions and discussion about a variety of topics related to their roles, responsibilities, personal goals, aspirations and progress. Peers tend to have something in common, whether it is membership of the same profession, membership of the same team (with members of different professions), membership of the same department or an interest in the same clinical specialty.

It can often seem less daunting to ask a question of a peer than to ask the same question of a manager. A peer relationship tends to be less threatening. There must be credibility and competence within the peer group, however, to avoid concerns about inadequate or wrong information. Peers also provide the encouragement needed for an individual to fulfil personal development goals, especially when the demands of a person's roles and goals are incompatible and cause tension. Everyone needs to be assured of their confidence to succeed in new roles and peer support can offer that reassurance.

Peer support groups can develop in many ways, serving as either formal or informal mechanisms for mutual support and development. Much peer support is to be found by attendance at conferences, workshops or special interest group meetings. Activities at local, regional or national level bring like-minded people together to learn with, and from, each other. Networking takes place and professional alliances are formed. These networks can often prove useful for research when the need arises. On a more informal basis, discussions might take place with a colleague or group of colleagues over coffee, lunch or a drink in the pub. The power of the informal peer support group should not be underestimated. More formal approaches might entail regular meetings with an agenda and designated chair. Peer group discussions might centre around the presentation and exploration of a case study, professional dilemma or concern. It might take the form of a journal club reviewing a paper, article or book of common interest. Any activity can provide the focus for peer learning and support. Peer learning can also provide the necessary amount of structure and discipline needed for individuals to commit themselves to achieving their learning objectives.

Collaborative learning

Collaborative learning can take many forms. For example, some learning might take place in a *learning set*. A learning set is composed of a small group of people, often from mixed disciplines, who commit to learning together and from each other. They meet periodically to discuss issues and challenges that they face, and from open discussion they gain insight into the experiences of the group (Perry, 1998). The learning set can thus act as both a learning and support mechanism.

A good deal of collaborative learning is likely to take place through some kind of project work where there are pre-defined goals and a timeframe for completion. The project is completed through collaborative effort where each person has something to contribute and where the learning for each person will be different to that of the others. Learning is likely to relate as much to the process of managing the task and the dynamics of the team as to gaining new information or using information in a different way. This kind of learning is still useful and worthy of note.

Where learning is structured, for example through courses organised by training departments or within institutes of higher education, seminars, tutorials or self-directed learning groups provide opportunities for debate and for learning through dialogue. Whatever the opportunity for sharing ideas and for working on joint ventures, collaborative learning has the advantage of structuring time and effort, pooling resources and of learning with other people for mutual benefit.

Learning independently

While there are many benefits to be gained from learning with other people either collaboratively or as a member of a group, sometimes there are times when this might not be possible, desirable or appropriate. Some people actually thrive by working and learning independently and they purposefully choose independent learning strategies. For some people, personal circumstances might make independent studies more convenient than alternative learning opportunities.

Activities such as portfolio development are most likely to be undertaken independently, as are reading and reviewing articles, papers or books or reflecting quietly on practice. Sharing thoughts with others and debating issues of common concern can enhance the learning that takes place, but independent learning can be more efficient when time is at a premium. More formally, one of the best known and best structured independent learning systems is the Open University which caters for independent learners from all backgrounds and circumstances. Within the system there are opportunities for shared learning through tutorials and, more selectively, through summer school, but independent learning is the dominant learning mode. Learning using technology and the internet is now becoming more common as individuals have greater access to personal computers.

Support from educators

Educators can often be a resource for individuals who are specialists in their own discipline but who have minimal knowledge of learning opportunities and educational processes. Educators have particular experience and expertise in relation to learning strategies and often in relation to research. Educators should therefore be able to provide advice, develop learning programmes and open up avenues of thinking about the potential of different situations to provide appropriate learning experiences.

Clinical supervisors/fieldwork educators

Supervisors of students of a profession tend to be the first line of support for those undertaking clinical placements. Supervisors have a particular remit that includes managing the placement, allocating and monitoring the caseload, facilitating learning, assessing the performance of the student and providing personal and professional support. Inevitably, there could be tensions between these areas of responsibility, but failure to support the student may lead to ineffective learning. Support for learning is thus paramount. Supervisors also have a duty to view fieldwork or clinical education as part of the process of life-long learning and to help ensure that the student's learning experience is a positive one. Hopefully, learning and professional development will continue to be addressed once the professional qualifying programme is complete. The supervisor can thus do much to encourage the student to record learning that takes place in the clinical setting in a way that might correlate with the requirements of a professional portfolio.

Developing the skills of the future workforce is a professional responsibility and crucial to the survival of the profession. However, the role and responsibilities of the clinical supervisor are often underestimated. The challenge is to be able to integrate clinical supervision with service provision. Support from the line manager is therefore crucial. Clinical supervision is normally an extension of an existing clinical role so any continuing professional development has to address both sets of responsibilities. In turn, learning can also arise from the supervisory process and its associated responsibilities.

Support from the professional body

Professional bodies have a number of responsibilities relating to the continuing professional development of their members, such as the following:

- Having a policy on continuing professional development.
- Monitoring environmental changes that affect practice and development needs.
- Researching, evaluating and supporting the implementation of changes in professional practice in response to society's changing demands.
- Promoting a culture of learning and continuing professional development within the profession.
- Supporting and guiding the membership in their endeavours to engage in continuing professional development.
- Maintaining standards through continuing professional development of members.
- Promoting relationships with providers of continuing professional education.
- Accrediting post-qualification programmes for continuing professional development.

The work of the profession, such as that described above, may be carried out by employees of the professional organisation but it is often supported by members of the profession who are drawn from different fields of practice and who represent different professional groups and interests. Making a contribution to the work of the professional body is a particular kind of learning activity that has benefits for the individual contributor and the profession as a whole. In essence, the profession makes provision for the support that other members need in developing their practice and expertise.

References

Burdett, J.O. (1994) To coach or not to coach, that is the question. In *Managing Learning* (C. Mabey & P. Iles, eds). Routledge, London.

Daloz, L. (1986) Effective teaching and mentoring. Cited in P. Jarvis (1995) *Adult and Continuing Education Theory and Practice*, 2nd edn. Routledge, London.

Department of Health (1998) *A First Class Service*. Department of Health, London.

Department of Health (1999) *Continuing Professional Development: Quality in the New NHS*. Department of Health, London.

Javernick, J.A. (1994) Professional growth through mentoring. *OT Week* 8 (24), 16–17.

Kalinauckas, P. (1995) Coaching for CPD. In *Continuing Professional Development – Perspectives on CPD in Practice* (S. Clyne, ed.). Kogan Page, London.

Megginson, D. & Pedlar, M. (1992) *Self-Development – A Facilitator's Guide*. McGraw Hill, Maidenhead.

Parsloe, E. (1995) *Coaching, Mentoring and Assessing: A Practical Guide to Developing Competence*. Kogan Page, London.

Perry, C. (1998) Why is CPD important for you now? Update. South Thames IHSM Briefing Issue 1 June 1998.

Chapter 13
Activities for Continuing Professional Development

Exercising choice

Throughout this book the emphasis has been on you taking control of your own continuing professional education and development to meet personal and career aspirations as well as statutory and service expectations. The breadth of opportunity for continuing professional development should not be under-estimated and in this final chapter many of the potential opportunities are outlined in order to remind you of the choice that is available.

It has been stressed that it is preferable that any professional development activity undertaken should be compatible with your learning style. Your personal circumstances may facilitate or hinder (even if temporarily) your ability to access education and development opportunities. However, opportunities are many and varied and in some ways opportunities have to be created. It is easy to think of the tried and tested, traditional methods of learning that have been used in the past. Now, however, there are many more openings and increased recognition of how learning takes place outside the academic environment. The Government is currently supporting work-based, experiential learning as a favoured mode of staff development. Institutes of higher education are becoming more flexible about accrediting (prior) experiential learning and in supporting individuals in different kinds of educational activity within the university, within the workplace and at home. No-one, whatever their circumstances, need now feel disadvantaged about gaining access to appropriate education and development experiences.

The following section presents a range of ideas for continuing professional development. It serves as a compendium of activities arranged in alphabetical order and cross-referenced as necessary. The nature of each activity is briefly outlined. More detail of the different activities may be found elsewhere in the book. Essentially, this chapter is intended to act as a point of reference to prompt ideas and thoughts about development opportunities. Whilst it is an extensive list, it is not exhaustive. You may find many more examples of learning opportunity. Hopefully, the principles of learning outlined elsewhere in the book will enable you to take advantage of any learning opportunities that arise and to present them in a way that shows evidence of your continuing professional development.

Activities for continuing professional development

Abstracts

Abstracts are often called for when papers or posters are to be presented at a conference. The abstract will be judged for its relevance to the conference and its intended audience and the paper or poster will be accepted or rejected on the merits of the abstract. An abstract has to be concise and focused so as to give essential information about the proposed presentation. Writing abstracts is a skill in itself and any that you prepare should be kept in your portfolio.

Acting up

Very occasionally opportunities arise for therapists to 'act up' into a higher grade position in the employing organisation pending recruitment to a post or whilst it is vacant, for example, for maternity or extended sick leave. There are often extra responsibilities attached to the job that attracts enhanced pay. The new role may afford opportunities to experience different facets of the work, for example, through extending clinical or management responsibilities, attending meetings or undertaking a different range of duties. Any experience like this can provide an opportunity for professional development. Reflections and learning from the experience can be recorded.

Action learning/action research

Action learning allows a team of people to address a problem on the job and to develop problem-solving strategies through team learning, ongoing discussion and feedback. This enables the work to be advanced in a direction that promotes desirable change within the organisation.

Adviser

Becoming an adviser implies that the individual has particular knowledge or expertise that others may want to learn and which the adviser is in a position to share. This may be because the individual has developed special skills or merely because he or she has greater knowledge than those seeking the advice. As an adviser, an individual may be called upon either within or beyond the employing organisation. The advice given will always need to reflect the context in which it is to be used. This means that the adviser must keep up to date in order to offer appropriate advice. Keeping skills and knowledge updated and advising others using this knowledge in their own situation is a CPD activity.

Agency work

Agency work offers the opportunity to work in a range of services on a short-term basis. Keeping abreast of current practice is essential so the maintenance of competence has to be a personal commitment. Each different work experience can be treated as a learning experience. New contexts of practice, new people and new systems all require adjustment and a degree of learning.

Appraisal

See performance review.

Articles: reading, reviewing and critically evaluating

One of the most common ways of updating and developing oneself professionally is by reading articles that are pertinent to professional work. Articles can be read just for information or for broadening personal knowledge and understanding, or they can be examined critically as part of a wider remit of evaluation and research. Reviewing articles for publication at the request of an editor is also a task that demands certain skills. Engaging in any of these activities can result in learning and professional development. A log should be kept of the articles that have been read or reviewed, with the date when the activity occurred. Any observations from reading can also be noted.
See also Publication.

Assessments

Carrying out assessments is fundamental to the work of any practitioner. The assessment process may relate to a particular practice model and will always reflect the service user's condition and circumstances. But there will be times when some of the circumstances are new and not encountered before. Perhaps a new form of assessment has to be undertaken with users who are normally assessed in another way, perhaps a practice model is being used for the first time, or perhaps a common assessment is being used with an individual with a very unusual condition or in particularly unusual circumstances. Methods and procedures may have to be adapted, measures may be difficult to ascertain or data interpretation may not be straightforward. Carrying out types of assessment that fall outside the norm can add to a practitioner's store of professional knowledge to be drawn upon again should the need arise. The assessment process, its circumstances, procedure, outcome and any personal observations are worth recording.

Audits

Auditing is one way of learning whether services are being delivered to the specifications and standards set. It is also a way for both individuals and teams to review service delivery in order to gain an understanding of strengths and limitations in the way services are provided. Taking a critical look at systems and processes can lead to lessons being learned and can help to identify where improvements might be made in the future.

Books

Writing books requires the author to undertake a certain amount of research activity to ensure currency and accuracy of information. The material has to be presented in a form that reflects the readership. Reading and writing skills are enhanced and reading books or consulting reference texts can add to personal knowledge.

Book reviews

Preparing a book review for an editor requires critical reading skills and an ability to present a concise, balanced appraisal of the published material. The topic of the book is likely to be of interest to the reviewer and as such it provides an opportunity to update, broaden or deepen knowledge of the subject.

Care pathways

Care pathways describe key events in the process of providing clinical care. They reflect the sequence and timing of interventions by different members of the clinical team. Preparing these pathways is a challenging activity that has to take account of many perspectives on care provision, the systems in place and the optimum levels of intervention for efficiency and effectiveness. Anyone who has prepared a care pathway will have learned a good deal from the process.

Case presentations

Making oral case presentations involves exploring a range of data on a given case and selecting and sequencing the material in order to present it to the audience in a meaningful way. The material needs to be sufficiently well understood so that any questions posed can be dealt with adequately, and this may involve additional research. It may also require reasoned arguments to be presented about intervention strategies and the theoretical basis for any actions that were taken or rejected.

Case studies

In a similar way to case presentations, the material pertinent to a given case (clinical or organisational) is researched and presented to an audience. It may be presented as a written document or as an oral case presentation. The case study will have been chosen because it is unusual or because it allows for the careful analysis and scrutiny of factors related to the case, so that lessons may be learned. Similar to case presentations, case studies demand research and the presentation of material in a logical sequence. The context of the case will need to be explored and cohesive arguments presented to substantiate judgements and courses of action taken.

Coaching

Coaching means working with an individual for whom there may be line management responsibilities in order to help the person to develop both personally and professionally in their job. There has to be a commitment both to teaching and to enabling learning so that the individual being coached can learn and grow. In some instances it might mean working and learning together where there are common challenges in the work situation.

Collaborative research

Collaborative research entails formalised work to address a given research problem (*see* Research). The advantage of working collaboratively is that several researchers work on the same study, pool their resources and support each other. The researchers become a 'learning community' (Reason, 1988), learning from each other in the research process. Collaborators may come from different parts of the service or from service and academic environments to carry out a study that is common to all.

Commissioned work

Anyone asked to undertake a project as a commission is usually perceived to have expertise in the relevant area. Each commission is likely to be unique in some or all of its features. Whilst commissioned work may involve drawing on existing knowledge and expertise, it may also involve researching new information or applying existing knowledge in a new way.

Committee membership or chairmanship

Serving on a committee can be an interesting and rewarding way of both contributing to developments and committee business and of broadening knowledge and skills. Focused discussions can lead to an enhanced understanding of the context of the work and of different perceptions of the issues raised and may result in improved problem-solving skills, especially where agenda items address new initiatives. Committee membership in any capacity, but particularly as chair, can lead to a greater understanding of the formalities of committee work and of the challenges of representing the views of others.

Computer-based interactive learning

This mode of learning is becoming increasingly popular with those who have difficulty accessing courses or educational programmes in other ways or where expertise is not readily available locally. For some people, computer learning may be the learning mode of choice as the potential of information technology is realised. Structured computer-based programmes require the student to interact with the computer by working step-by-step through exercises. The programme assesses the merits of the student's answer and either progresses to more advanced levels incrementally in line with the student's developing knowledge or revisits the knowledge base to ensure that basic knowledge is grasped before the student moves on to the next step.

Conferences

New skills and knowledge can arise from both planning and attending conferences. Planning conferences demands research and organisational skills; attending conferences requires active listening, sometimes active participation, and always critical thinking and reflection about the material presented. Learning is reinforced where an assessment is made of the potential use and application of any new knowledge to the work or situation in which the participant is normally involved.

Consultancy

Consultancy demands high levels of knowledge and skills, usually to expert levels. However, learning and professional development can occur as expertise is applied to new situations and contexts locally, nationally or internationally. Often some research is required.

Courses

Courses present one of the most favoured ways of gaining exposure to new material and new thinking. However, attendance is not enough. Active participation, reflection on learning, identification of personal learning outcomes and evaluation of the potential use of the new learning will enable individuals to gain the most from the course as a learning experience.

Critical incidents

Critical incidents are seen as turning points where outcomes are either good or bad. Lessons can be learned from gaining a full understanding of a critical incident, and the sequence of events that led up to it that influenced the outcome. Lessons can be learned from incidents that led to both positive and negative outcomes.

Critical reviews

Critically reviewing an activity or written material requires the reviewer to engage with what is being done or said and to draw out the strengths and limitations of the material and the way it is presented, in a manner that is consistent and fair. A critical review requires some judgements to be made about the relative merits of the material but those judgements must be substantiated with evidence rather than merely opinion. Critical reviews can be undertaken of books, articles, literature, workshops, conferences, or any other learning experience.

Debates

Engaging in debate can often mean thinking on your feet to present views and examples of experiences that might contribute to others' understanding of the topic. Engaging in debate also requires active listening skills to follow the arguments and to challenge them where appropriate. Learning can take place through any preparations undertaken for the debate and from being exposed to others' views.

Designs

See Plans.

Diaries, logs, critical reflections

Recording critical reflections on events is useful. Thinking about and planning what to write is probably the most useful activity of all because this focuses attention on what has been experienced and helps to develop the insights that evolve into new learning. A commitment to writing down personal reflections (and not just descriptions) ensures a thorough evaluation of the issues. Often the experience of recording insights in a diary or log leads to the emerging of new insights. A record of the reflections will provide an archive of material that shows how personal perceptions arise and change over time.

Distance learning

Distance learning involves following a structured programme of learning away from the academic setting. The programme may be pre-set by an academic institution or established by the learner and agreed by the institution from where support and guidance may be given. Support may come from a programme of face-to-face tutorials, telephone support, on-line support or through peer group meetings arranged locally.

Doctoral studies

A select few individuals will feel able to be challenged by studies leading to a PhD or taught doctorate. Registration with a university is essential. Supervisors will provide the academic support, particularly where the programme is totally research-based, but essentially, doctoral studies involve independent study. Doctoral students will need to show that they have mastery of the field of study and that they can make a unique contribution to the knowledge base in the field. Doctoral studies are normally completed over four to six years part time so motivation and commitment are essential.

Education and higher education

As with doctoral studies, some individuals wish to go on after initial professional qualification to achieve higher academic awards through continuing professional education. Structured postgraduate studies that lead to a master's degree are the most popular. An increasing number of health professionals are following postgraduate studies for their own interest and personal satisfaction. The academic award provides the goal. The dissertation may address a work or profession-related issue so that the studies have a direct bearing on career development, as well as enhancing the practitioner's knowledge base.

Evening classes

Relevant education can sometimes be pursued out of work hours through evening classes. Some classes may not be specifically planned for health practitioners but nevertheless fulfil a need for personal or professional development. Learning a second language would be an example.

Exhibitions or displays

Preparing an exhibition or display can involve a surprisingly large amount of work. Some of this work may involve research about the topic or about the audience in order to present the most appropriate material in the most appropriate way.

Higher degrees

See Education and Doctoral studies

Independent studies

Independent studies can be approached in at least two ways: through learning contracts (see later) that are agreed and managed in the workplace, or through university accredited independent learning modules or units of study. Both expect the learner to set the agenda for learning and manage the identified action plan. The benefits are that there is a clear goal to be achieved, the learning activity can be planned exactly to reflect the learner's needs, it can be carried out in the workplace if necessary, it is structured within a known timeframe, and is supported through a network of people agreed at the outset. One main disadvantage is that independent learning is just that, learning without peer group support. The learner is the only one following that particular programme.

Information leaflets

Health care practitioners are frequently required to prepare information leaflets for patients, carers and other service users. Accurate, concise information has to be given in terms that the reader can readily understand. Research is needed about both the topic and the readership in order to present the right information.

In-house education and training

Some very valuable education programmes can be provided for staff in-house. These can range from one-off lunchtime presentations to a programme lasting several months. Professional development can occur through both organising and participating in the events. In-house sessions provide opportunities for interprofessional education and team learning.

Inventions

Occasionally, health professionals are in the position of having to address clinical or functional problems by inventing something new because there is nothing commercially available that is suitable. Learning takes place through problem-solving and from bringing together a range of information and resources from disparate areas of medicine, science and technology. The research, problems encountered, solutions found and evaluation of the end-product can all be important learning experiences to record for personal use, and they could be published for the wider community.

Jobswaps

Arranging and taking part in a jobswap for a time-limited period can help practitioners to use existing knowledge and skills in a new area of practice and to develop contextual knowledge pertinent to the new situation. It provides a format for maintaining and developing competence and expertise across services and agencies locally, nationally or even internationally.

Journal club

Journal clubs bring together people, sometimes across professions and disciplines, who share an interest in learning through reading and debate. Journal articles are critically evaluated and the relative merits of the contents are evaluated. The different perspectives presented by participants add to the learning process.

Learning contracts

Working with a learning contract can formalise learning and provide an agreed structure for exploring issues of personal interest that may not be reflected in any other educational programme. The learning topic or goal is unique to the learner and the way in which the learning process is defined is also unique, tailored to meet individual needs. Most of the learning is likely to be experiential, underpinned by some theoretical work to set the context for learning and enhance understanding. The learning plan is recorded, formally agreed with a mentor and is completed within an agreed timescale. See Anderson *et al.* (1996) for further information.

Learning sets

Learning sets bring people together for a particular purpose with an agenda for learning from and with each other. Group members will share the same interest and want to use the peer group as a learning resource. Learning sets depend on active participation and dialogue. The group manages itself and meets on a regular basis to discuss commonly agreed topics or to share perspectives. The nature of the learning can often result in personal development. Commitment to the learning set is essential.

Lectures

Attending lectures is one of the more traditional ways of being exposed to information and ideas. However, lectures are only successful as a tool for learning if those in attendance are active listeners. Reflecting on the material presented can enhance the learning that has taken place and thinking creatively about the future use of new knowledge can help to ensure that learning becomes meaningful.

Lecturing

Preparing and presenting lectures can also be a way of learning. Material has to be thoroughly researched, sifted, selected and organised into a logical presentation designed specifically for the lecture audience. Audiovisual resources to support the lecture have to be prepared and used effectively. Knowledge and presentation skills are thus developed.

Lecture tours

A lecture tour involves researching and preparing for a series of lectures. The process (*see* Lecturing) can be quite demanding but often there are hidden benefits such as sharing expert knowledge with an attentive audience in a new context. Engaging the audience and encouraging questions may offer new perspectives on the lecture topic.

Lecturer practitioner

Lecturer practitioner posts in various professions are becoming increasingly popular. They present an opportunity to mix practice and academic duties and normally involve responsibility for facilitating the learning of student practitioners. Coaching students is often a two-way learning process. Teaching and coaching skills need to be developed and competence in practice must be maintained.

Legal work

Medico-legal work is a growing area of practice for some professions. Apart from being a competent, experienced and able practitioner who may have particular expertise in a given field of practice, the practitioner also has to develop knowledge and understanding of legal processes and the skills to present written statements for the court and give verbal evidence in court.

Literature searches

Literature searches are normally done for a specific purpose to seek information about what other people have done in the field. Literature searches may support projects, evidence-based practice or research. They require knowledge of how to access data bases and other sources of literature and how to review literature critically. They are demanding of time and energy but can reveal new information which can be appraised for its relevance to practice.

Management and management training

Taking on management responsibilities adds another dimension to practice. Management tends initially to be at an operational level but progression may lead to responsibility for the strategic direction of the service. Health practitioners also have greater opportunities now for moving into general management and for taking overarching responsibility for the coordination of a range of services and the management of a number of different professionals. Apart from the management of people there is often responsibility for financial management. Education and training in management techniques and strategies can help but much learning is done on the job and emerges through experience. It is worthwhile keeping records of personal strategies that have been successful in the management arena.

Master classes

Master classes provide opportunities for learning from experts in small seminar groups or through one-to-one interaction. Master classes are probably not as well used as they might be. For those who are participating or for those who have to prepare and give the class, the demands involved can provide meaningful learning experiences.

Master's degree studies

A significant number of health professionals who hold a bachelor's degree pursue Master's level studies at some stage in their career. They want the intellectual challenges that higher education can provide and they want to feel as if they have mastery of some element of their work. They may undertake this level of study as preparation for a career move, perhaps into education or management. Most health professionals have the capacity for attaining a Master's degree if they wish. The process, however, is more important than the end product as it can entail significant personal and professional growth. Satisfaction after graduation often comes from finding a way in which new-found knowledge and skills can be used in practice.

Mentoring

Mentoring is primarily a support mechanism for individuals to assist them in their professional development. Mentors should consider the additional skills required in the role and take steps to attain the necessary knowledge that will help them to be successful. The development of appropriate skills is a learning responsibility; facilitating learning and professional development in others is a learning opportunity.

Networking

There are many opportunities as a health practitioner to meet with colleagues in formal and informal situations to discuss areas of mutual interest. Networking is very important. Sometimes new information emerges immediately from discussions, at other times discussions provide cues to new information that are followed up later. The most important aspect of networking is the opportunity to exchange contact information so that enquiries can be pursued later. Learning about other people's experiences is an excellent way of sharing and validating ideas.

Paper presentations

Preparing and presenting papers at conferences makes demands but also provides an opportunity to share work with others, hear other people's questions and observations about the paper, and gain new insights through their views on the material presented.

Peer learning and development groups

Meeting with peers within your service or from other services can provide support and opportunities for sharing and working with new ideas. Peer groups can act as reference groups to help practitioners to discover new information and to validate learning and new proposals for practice.

Performance review

Some kind of informal, or preferably formal, performance review is essential if education, training and development needs are to be identified. All health professionals are expected to have appraisals or performance reviews and personal development plans in place that identify education and training needs and the ways in which they will be met.

PhD

See Doctoral studies.

Photographs

Sometimes evidence of continuing professional development can be hard to collect because of the nature of the activity. A series of photographs taken to illustrate professional development activity or to show how new learning has been implemented can provide a way of supporting written records of experiential learning.

Pilot studies

Resources to explore or support new initiatives can be hard to come by. Sometimes an idea or initiative is itself too big to address all in one go. Pilot studies provide a means of working on an aspect of the proposal so that it can be evaluated to determine whether a larger project should go ahead. A focused, systematic pilot study in a defined area of practice can support both service and professional development.

Plans

Plans or designs can form evidence of continuing professional development if they represent a scheme for an innovation that a practitioner has created. These would normally be supported by a script which sets the plans into context and shows how they relate to new learning or professional development.

Poster presentations

Poster presentations provide a visual means of explaining an innovation in practice or in service delivery. Professional conferences often provide the opportunity to present posters. Preparing a good poster makes significant demands in terms of research, collation and selection of relevant material and of presenting ideas in a visual way that captures and sustains the attention of an audience. The poster and any written material prepared as a supporting handout are evidence of continuing professional development.

Postgraduate study

Many universities now offer a whole range of opportunities for health professionals to study after their initial graduation and registration. Postgraduate studies do not necessarily require registration for a complete programme leading to a higher academic award. Many postgraduate studies are now offered on a modular basis where a single module can be taken independently as a means of professional development. (*See also* Doctoral studies, Master's degrees.)

Presentations: case studies, conference papers, posters

All presentations demand research, selection and organisation of material for the needs of a particular audience. This obviously requires judgement about what is appropriate and how it can be best presented. Audio-visual material has to be prepared to support the presentation. Presentation skills have to be honed and refined and questions have to be anticipated. The whole experience is demanding but can generate new learning in a variety of forms. (*See also* Case studies, Paper presentations, Poster presentations.)

Private practice

In order to keep up-to-date with changes in practice, self employed practitioners or those engaged in private practice must engage in various types of learning, particularly in their specialist area of work. It is extremely important for private practitioners to ensure that these learning experiences are recorded to demonstrate ongoing competence in the area of practice.

Professional activities: committee work, working groups

From time to time, a practitioner may be involved in work that reflects the needs of a professional or statutory regulatory body. This becomes personal learning activity, especially if it is ground-breaking work, even though it may primarily be for somebody else. Learning that emerges from service on professional and other committees is worthy of note, as is the consideration of the application of new knowledge in practice.

Projects

Project work takes many forms and the multiple activities undertaken to support it often require the processing of both existing and new material in different ways. New insights tend to arise from manipulating data, even if the project is small and time-limited. These insights need to be captured, not just for the project, but also as part of a reflective log.

Project group membership

Projects may be undertaken collaboratively as part of a process of service evaluation or development. Not only are the benefits of project work applicable, so is the fact that learning can arise from group membership. This is particularly so if the group comprises representatives of other professions or agencies. Learning can take many forms and need not be limited to discovering new facts. Being a group member and working together may also provide valuable learning experience.

Protocols

Protocols can take two forms: research protocols and protocols as a blueprint for practice. The first is a formal plan or proposal for a piece of research which must be carefully prepared. It is normally a concisely written plan that sets the proposed research into the context of what is already known about the topic and details the methods by which the study will be carried out (Drummond, 1996).

A protocol is usually devised by and for a group of professionals setting the parameters of a treatment process in a defined area of practice. Writing it presents challenges in terms of reasoning and decision-making to establish the structure and content of the protocol. It becomes a reference point for common, best practice (Hopkins & Smith, 1993).

Public speaking

Apart from making presentations at conferences or giving lectures to peers, public speaking could include any event that involves being in the public eye and where information is presented to an audience. It might involve giving a talk to service users or carers, to voluntary groups or organisations, or at careers evenings or similar events. It might also include radio or television broadcasts. The research and preparation for the event has to address the needs of the audience.

Publication

It is important to disseminate research findings and to share examples of good practice. Preparing articles or reports for publication means writing succinctly in a well-organised way about practice activity or concepts. It is vital that the report is unbiased and, where appropriate, for the paper to be grounded in literature and for findings to be based on evidence. Preparing material for publication is a skill in itself, but the end result provides good evidence of CPD.

Quality assurance initiatives

Any quality assurance initiative is usually underpinned by a desire to learn and to improve practice. Setting standards, auditing services and implementing changes all aid quality improvement and contribute to learning.

Reading

Continuing professional development can take many forms, but reading is likely to be the activity in which most practitioners engage at some time or another. Reading can simply be for interest. However, reading with a clear agenda that involves a systematic, structured process of seeking information, actively making comparisons with other texts, or formulating a critique of the work can enhance learning. An agenda helps to focus the reading and encourages active participation with the work.

Reports

Preparing reports for an audience means assembling a carefully selected range of information and presenting it in written form. The report is normally about an initiative or activity previously undertaken, possibly where conclusions have been drawn and recommendations made for subsequent action. Careful attention has to be paid to making points clearly and concisely, backed up by relevant arguments and discussion. Reports provide evidence of work undertaken.

Research (action, case study, collaborative, descriptive, illuminative research)

Any research associated with practice or service delivery will constitute activity through which learning occurs. The essence of research is to update knowledge, to assess current knowledge in new contexts or to develop a knowledge base. There are many different approaches to research and any will lead to learning, not just about practice but also about the research process.

Sabbatical

An individual offered a sabbatical is able to take leave from employment to pursue a project of special interest, normally associated with, or complementary to, his or her normal work. The experience will not only result in learning but it will also have relevance to the individual's employment because new learning can be applied back in the workplace.

Secondments

Being seconded to another service, or to a different part of the service, provides an opportunity to complement knowledge and to view service delivery from another perspective. It is often possible to see relationships that were not obvious before and to propose initiatives that enhance collaborative practice.

Self-directed learning

Self-directed learning covers all aspects of learning and professional development that are initiated and/or carried out independently. It requires learners to be well motivated and resourceful and to have a commitment to meeting learning goals. Both pre-set and new learning outcomes can be achieved.

Service developments

Service developments arise out of policy changes or audit activity that indicate the need for new ways of providing services. Changes need to be grounded in research that indicates why and how change is needed. Some staff development may be necessary to support the initiative.

Service evaluation and review

Service evaluation, especially one undertaken systematically or though audit, may lead to new insights about service provision and to recommendations for service development and change. Lessons learned from one review may be applicable elsewhere.

Skill development

Whatever the knowledge, skills or expertise needed for professional practice, there is always room for improvement and development. Additional qualifications in areas such as counselling can be sought, advanced technical skills involving equipment or personal techniques can be developed to support progression to a more specialised post or area of practice, or enhanced practical skills may promote role extension. It is important to document the learning and changes in professional performance that take place through skill enhancement and development.

Special interest group activity

Practitioners who have special expertise or interest in a field of practice tend to form networks with people who have similar interests and skills. Groups of people who communicate regularly on specialist topics have the opportunity to learn from one another. Communication may be informal (conversations, email) or may be through formalised group activity at a local, regional or national level. Workshops and conferences provide an opportunity for sharing experiences and new knowledge. Presenting conference papers can involve significant research and the ability to select and organise material appropriately. Case presentations can also provide a medium for sharing expertise. Special interest group activity presents wide-ranging means of keeping abreast of practice, taking stock of one's own practice in relation to that of others in the same field, and for maintaining competence. Selected, relevant learning from these activities can be logged in a CPD portfolio.

Staff development programmes: organising, leading, attending

Staff development programmes are primarily established to address a learning need for an individual or a group of staff. Attending such events has obvious benefits, especially if consolidated through reflection and later application of new knowledge in practice. Organising and leading development programmes requires research, preparation and presentation and the resultant learning is likely to be different to that of participants. Exposure to development programmes can be beneficial, but participation in debate, wherever this is possible, involves active learning which may be longer lasting.

Standard setting and monitoring

Any activity to improve service quality can only enhance learning and understanding about the strengths and limitations of areas of practice. Standard setting involves breaking down practice into activity that is auditable and assessing it against previously-documented standards that are desirable and achievable. Current practice is monitored and assessed so that areas needing improvement can be identified. These are inevitably learning activities that may have implications personally or at team or organisational level.

Student supervision

Many practitioners enjoy the challenges of enabling student learning. Those practitioners who can engage openly in discussions and acknowledge their own learning needs as part of the agenda tend to gain more from the experience of supervising students than those that cannot. It can be quite empowering to have a peer relationship with students where supervisor and student learn from each other.

Study tours

A study tour set up with a particular agenda for learning can be very rewarding. It may involve visits arranged locally, nationally or internationally. It is important to set goals before embarking on a tour as time goes very fast and it is easy to get distracted and fail to meet the aims of the study. Reflections on how goals were met will serve as an aid to learning.

Supervision: professional, research, project

Both giving and receiving supervision can be a learning experience. Preparation for receiving supervision is crucial as it means that some thought has been given to the agenda. The discussions can then be focused and are likely to lead to better use of time and outcomes that are useful to both parties. Supervision in the workplace tends to be a line management activity and may set the scene for personal development plans in relation to service need and professional development. Research or project supervision is time-limited and task-oriented, but significant learning can ensue.

Teaching

Anyone who takes responsibility for teaching, whether it involves providing clinical education, in-service education or sessional lecturing, will need to be up to date with subject content and with teaching and learning methods. Often a significant amount of research and preparation is involved in order to present a coherent and well thought out educational package. This can require the teacher to update his or her own practice in order to be sure of presenting the most up to date information. The educational programme should be based on evidence of best practice. New learning may arise through the research and preparation that is carried out, and through the process of teaching itself.

Team learning

Learning with people who commonly work together, whether in a uniprofessional or interprofessional team, can have benefits. The work can be shared, different perspectives can be aired and each member can learn from the others. Provided that each member plays a part, team learning can enable members to function significantly better, both as a team and in relation to the service they provide.

Videos

Videos can provide pictorial evidence of working with, or on behalf of, service users or of learning situations in which an individual has participated. It is helpful to have some written material to supplement the video to set the context for the activity. A short reflective report can often clarify the learning that has emerged.

Visits: local, national, international

Visits have enormous potential for learning. Although some learning may take place when a visit is carried out spontaneously, more focused learning can take place if preparations are made for the visit and an agenda is set for what is to be explored. In either case, reflections after the visit can aid the learning process.

Voluntary work

Any voluntary work carried out outside working hours may provide an opportunity for learning that can help to develop supplementary knowledge and skills relevant to employment as a health care practitioner. Learning need not be confined to on-the-job activity or formal education directly associated with employment but can embrace a range of activities that take place beyond the work environment.

Working groups

Working groups are often set up for a limited period to address a problem or work on a project. Each group member may have a particular remit so that activity is shared and new knowledge is pooled to help the problem-solving process. Exposure to the project activity and discussions with other group members can provide the forum for new learning and professional development.

Writing articles, papers, reports, books, information leaflets

Most practitioners engage in writing as part of their everyday work. Some projects make more demands than others but most require some research to be carried out. Material has to be selected, sequenced and prepared appropriately for the readership. Whatever is written may be suitable as evidence of continuing professional development.

References

Anderson, G., Boud, D. & Sampson, J. (1996) *Learning Contracts: A Practical Guide.* Kogan Page, London.

Drummond, A. (1996) *Research Methods for Therapists.* Chapman and Hall, London.

Hopkins, H. & Smith, H. (eds) (1993) *Willard and Spackman's Occupational Therapy*, 8th edn. Lippincott, Philadelphia.

Reason, P. (ed.) (1988) *Human Enquiry in Action: Developments in New Paradigm Research.* Sage Publications, London.

Realising Dreams

Continuing professional development is primarily to do with you as a person. There may be statutory requirements for you to maintain and demonstrate ongoing professional competence, there may be professional expectations of you to ensure that you are capable of offering 'best practice' in the current health care climate, but at the end of the day you have expectations of yourself so that you will continue along the road of life-long learning and seek out opportunities for continuing professional development. It is your career, your professional journey and you are in control of it. You need to find the most appropriate route for achieving your goals.

Initial professional education provides the foundation on which to build, but each person has different strengths and different aspirations. You need to be able to recognise your talents, develop them and use them to their full potential. In order to do this you need to set out your goals, to develop your capacity for learning and to organise yourself so that continuing professional development becomes an integral feature of professional life. In this way you work at taking steps to simultaneously maintain competence in your job, develop competence and skills for the next career move, and work towards longer term career goals.

It is important that you aim for more than just the minimum professional development to get by. Continuing professional development can be flexible, is wide-ranging and offers something for everyone, but it needs to be well thought out – it needs a plan. Continuing professional education is one aspect of continuing professional development that will suit those who want to be stretched and stimulated by the academic challenges that higher education offers. Making space for and finding resources to support university education can be difficult but the benefits outweigh the costs and are worth striving for.

Look after yourself in the process. Learning and development activity always make personal demands and demands on family life. Do not let continuing professional development take over your life; it should be an integral part of your practice and should become a way of supporting you on your professional journey. Do maintain a balance of activity that will allow you to achieve your goals in the most enjoyable way.

Continuing professional development and continuing professional education open up new avenues for learning, new ways of thinking and new career paths. These are all aspects of a professional journey that is unique to you. It is up to you to seek out and take advantage of CPD opportunities. Make sure that you take time to understand what learning has taken place as a result of these opportunities and that you record it appropriately. Do not hide your achievements away, be proud of what you have done. If you have found ways of continuing your professional development successfully then make sure that you help others to do the same. Take steps to engage others in continuing professional development, to strengthen them, to support them on their professional journey and to help them realise their dreams.

Index